THE
FREEDIET®

*A Clinically Proven Plan to Heal Your Gut and
Thyroid and Free Yourself from Pain, Fatigue,
Fogginess, and Fat*

DR. TOM ROFRANO

The FreeDiet®

Copyright 2019 by Thomas Rofrano

All rights reserved. No part of this book may be used or reproduced in any manner whatsoever without the written permission of the author except for brief quotations embodied in articles and reviews.

This book provides information to help you achieve optimal health and should be used to supplement rather than replace the advice of your doctor or health professional. It should not be considered a treatment or cure for any disease. If you know or suspect you have a health condition or have persistent symptoms, it is recommended that you seek your physician's advice. Extensive efforts were made to ensure the information in this book was accurate at publication date. The author and publisher disclaim liability for any outcomes that may occur from following the methods described in this book. The case studies in this book are actual patients of the author, some of whose names have been changed to protect their privacy.

The following statement applies to any dietary supplements mentioned in this book: This statement has not been evaluated by the FDA. This product is not intended to diagnose, treat, cure, or prevent any disease.

Identifiers:
ISBN 978-1-7331898-1-1 (paperback)
ISBN 978-1-7331898-0-4 (digital)
Library of Congress Control Number: 2019914248
Edition 1.0

Dr. Tom Rofrano
2401 PGA Blvd Ste 132
Palm Beach Gardens, FL 33410
drtomrofrano.com

FREE GIFTS FOR YOU

See nmcwellness.com/FreeDietGifts to receive the following PDF's to help you follow along and track your success with the FreeDiet®.

The FreeDiet® Phase 1 Food Chart
The FreeDiet® Phase 1 Shopping List
The FreeDiet® Phase 1 14-Day Sample Meal Plan

The FreeDiet® Health Goals and Health Assessment Quiz
The FreeDiet® Progress Chart

DEDICATION

To my dad, Douglas Rofrano, MD, who initially sparked my interest in health care.

To my mom, Jeannie Lochner, RN, for steering me in the direction of natural health.

To my wife, Dawn, a beautiful person, an amazing cook, who has been at my side for 27 years.

To my daughter, Adriana, who has inspired me to raise my level of contribution to this world.

CONTENTS

INTRODUCTION

It all started when I was 12 years old, and my mom brought me with her to this new place in town called a health food store. Little did I know that my life was about to change forever. The bottles of vitamins, powders, and elixirs fascinated me. While my mother quickly ran her errand, I scoured through the nutrition pamphlets and books, amazed. Looking back, it felt like I was walking through the wardrobe in *The Chronicles of Narnia*.

I brought home a brochure on all the vitamins and minerals and their effects on the body. I must have read it a hundred times. You mean you can improve your health with something as simple as vitamins? My father was a medical doctor, so all I knew up until that point were the medications I was given when I was sick or injured—which was admittedly quite often and never actually getting better.

My mom soon returned to the store and brought home the book *Let's Get Well* by Adelle Davis. I read it cover to cover. For the first time, I realized that by changing your diet, you could dramatically improve your health.

That started me on a quest for reading and learning as much as I could about health, fitness, and nutrition. I wanted to know two things:

1. Why was I always getting sick and injured?
2. How can I fix it?

Those two questions are with me to this day and directed towards how I can help others.

Why are you sick (as in what is the root cause), and *how can you get better* (as in real solutions)?

So many people are feeling unwell these days. Tired, aches and pains, overweight, brain fog, headaches, digestive and skin issues, thyroid conditions, insomnia, and then the resulting anxiety and depression because you're feeling so terrible and constantly wondering what's wrong. All the doctors say your tests are fine—it's stress, or your four kids, or what do you expect, you're entering menopause. They often suggest medication for depression or anxiety and send you on your way, frustrated with no answers.

Would you like to be free of all this?

With the FreeDiet®, you can become free of pain, fatigue, fogginess, and fat. You can heal your gut and thyroid. You can free yourself from this misery and feel the best you have in years—we're talking vibrant health!

The FreeDiet® is a diet that is free of foods most commonly responsible for inflammation, digestive, and other chronic health issues. It's not only gluten free, but it's free of gluten, grains, sugar, yeast, dairy, eggs, soy, legumes, nightshades, and processed foods.

The FreeDiet® incorporates the best of the elimination diet, Candida diet, Paleo, and Autoimmune Paleo. It's low in histamines and oxalates and can have ketogenic effects as well.

I created and refined the FreeDiet® through successfully seeing over 100,000 patients visits during the last 33-plus years at my Natural Medicine Clinic in Palm Beach Gardens, Florida. However, I originally created this for myself. I was suffering from all the above symptoms plus Hashimoto's and rheumatoid arthritis, and I needed a way to heal myself. None of the other diets or protocols were working. The FreeDiet®, however, worked.

Some of the health issues I have seen improve or completely resolve in patients following the FreeDiet® include:

- Digestive issues: bloating, gas, pain, indigestion, reflux, heartburn, IBS, IBD, colitis, diarrhea, and constipation
- Fatigue
- Brain Fog (lack of focus, concentration, and/or memory)
- Excess fat: weight loss resistance
- Pain: neck, back, joint, and muscle pain
- Anxiety
- Depression
- Insomnia
- Vertigo
- Headaches
- Migraines
- Sinus congestion
- Tinnitus
- Hashimoto's autoimmune thyroid
- Graves' disease (hyperthyroidism)
- Thyroid nodules and goiter
- High blood pressure
- High cholesterol and triglycerides
- High blood sugar (diabetes)
- Iron overload/high ferritin
- Parasites: blastocystis hominis and others
- Candida/yeast overgrowth
- Dysbiosis (bacterial overgrowth)
- Leaky gut (increased intestinal permeability)
- Skin conditions: acne, eczema, psoriasis, rashes, rosacea, lichen sclerosus, dandruff, itchy skin and scalp
- Hair loss (alopecia)
- Autoimmune conditions including lupus, multiple sclerosis, scleroderma, nephropathy (kidney disease), vasculitis, autoimmune hepatitis
- Rheumatoid arthritis
- Gout
- Numbness and tingling/peripheral neuropathy
- Chronic UTIs
- Interstitial cystitis
- PCOS, infertility, PMS
- Fibrocystic breasts
- Low testosterone
- Poor wound healing
- Immune system weakness (low WBCs)

How can one diet help with all these conditions?

Inflammation is an underlying cause of most chronic health conditions. The FreeDiet® lowers inflammation, as evidenced by pre- and post-lab tests on countless patients. The following are the reasons why this works.

First, The FreeDiet® is free of the most common food allergens and sensitivities which can cause numerous symptoms. Being free of gluten and grains, in particular, has been linked to significantly reduced inflammation in the body. Dairy, eggs, and soy are also common allergens. Legumes, which can be very difficult to digest, have been linked to digestive issues and leaky gut. Nightshades are a class of foods that have been shown to cause inflammation in certain individuals, especially those with autoimmune conditions. Finally, processed foods and Genetically Modified Organisms (GMOs) are eliminated due to their adverse and inflammatory effects on the gut and entire body.

Second, the FreeDiet® is low in sugar and carbohydrates, thus driving the body to burn excess fat for fuel and lower high blood sugar, triglycerides, cholesterol, and inflammation while balancing hormones.

Third, since the FreeDiet® is free of gluten, grains, sugar, and yeast, it has within it the Candida/yeast diet and helps balance your microbiome. This can heal leaky gut and chronic digestive and skin problems caused by yeast, bacteria, or parasites since they all thrive on sugar.

Fourth, the FreeDiet® is high in fresh vegetables, fiber, nutrients, and essential fats, all of which help with reducing inflammation and detoxifying heavy metals and other toxins.

Fifth, proper nutritional supplementation can support all the body systems, create a healthy immune and inflammatory response, and provide more energy and mental clarity.

Before you get started, the FreeDiet® works best if you can commit to following it 100 percent for the first 28 days. If you are going to cheat occasionally or not do it all the way, you will likely not get the amazing results you're looking for. On the other hand, if you can commit and follow the FreeDiet® as outlined in this book, I am sure it will be well worth the effort, and you can feel the best you have in years!

Patient success stories on the FreeDiet®:

- Ellen, a 56-year-old woman, was able to resolve her autoimmune condition within three months, clear up her fatigue, insomnia, brain fog, migraines, vertigo, joint pain, chronic constipation, and is feeling like a new person—the best she's felt in years!
- Janelle, a 36-year-old woman, was able to shrink her 4-plus cm thyroid nodule by 73 percent, as well as resolving her fatigue, brain fog, headaches, digestive issues, and weight loss resistance after three months on the FreeDiet®. During this time, she dropped 23 pounds!
- Terry, a 46-year-old woman, was able to shrink her 4 cm thyroid nodule by 30 percent, resolve her fatigue, dizziness, tinnitus, brain fog, anxiety, headaches, insomnia, pain, digestive symptoms, hair loss, shortness of breath, and anemia in her first three months. She lost 15 pounds in six weeks.
- Tom, a 61-year-old man, was able to resolve his fatigue, neuropathy, dizziness, shortness of breath, back and joint pain. Within four weeks, he decreased his blood pressure 35 points and cholesterol 65 points, both down to normal, and raised his testosterone 227 points to optimal levels. He did this without medication and lost 11 pounds in that first month.
- Jasmine, a 62-year-old woman, was able to resolve her chronic knee pain, numbness and tingling, headaches, vertigo, insomnia, fatigue, digestive issues, and balance her thyroid. She lost 12 pounds in the first two months, and since then has lost a total of 28 pounds, achieving her desired weight.

These are just a few of the thousands of patients who have experienced the benefits of the FreeDiet®. Once you read and follow the FreeDiet®, you too can become free of pain and misery, enjoy vibrant health, and feel the best you have in years! I'm looking forward to your success.

CHAPTER 1

My Story and How it Can Help You

People have often said to me, "Well, this diet is easy for you because you are so healthy, disciplined, and in shape." What most people don't realize is that I absolutely know what it's like to feel sick, miserable, and unhealthy.

I was sick a lot when I was a child. You would think otherwise since my father was a medical doctor and my mother was a nurse. Of course, we had plenty of medication available for us six kids. That's right; my mom had six children in eight years. It was pretty crazy around our house. But despite it all, I had a constant stuffy nose and frequent sore throats. After multiple rounds of antibiotics and allergy medication, I had to have my tonsils surgically removed at age seven. That was just the beginning.

I had rosacea, and the other kids in school would make fun of my red, blotchy face. I had bumps on the back of my arms, also known as chicken skin, as well as frequent canker sores, bedwetting, nosebleeds, OCD, dandruff, athlete's foot, acne, and warts on my hands, feet, and even my face.

I went to so many different doctors, all of whom knew my father. I used to go to the podiatrist at age 13 weekly to have a huge plantar wart that seemed the size of a quarter scraped, cut, and gouged out of my heel. In between visits, I had to put stinging acid on the wart.

This went on for months, and the wart still didn't clear up. Every week I would wait well over an hour before he would even see me. After I got tortured, I would have to limp home for three miles.

That's not all. I had irritable bowel syndrome (IBS), so every day before school, I would be on the toilet for what seemed like an eternity, having four or five bowel movements before 8 AM. I would then have to run almost a mile, in my school uniform, just to make it to school on time. Many days I would arrive embarrassingly late.

I was the shortest boy in eighth grade. At age 13, I entered high school at 4'11" and 98 pounds. I didn't start growing facial hair until my senior year. I was too short to make the high school basketball team, my number one love, and too small to even try out for football, so I joined the track team.

This only made things worse. I had neck pain, mid and low back pain, sprained ankles, sprained wrists, chest/sternum/rib pain, shoulder pain, hip pain, knee pain, shin splints, and plantar fasciitis during my time running track. The only treatments were whirlpools and tape—thick, white, sticky tape. I had almost every part of my body taped at one time or another, which did not help at all.

With each injury, I had to take more time off from track practice, which kept me from reaching my lofty aspirations: winning gold in the Olympics and setting three world records in the long jump, triple jump, and high jump.

Just before my senior year, my coach was told by a university coach and two college standouts that despite all my health issues and injuries, I had the most potential of anyone on the team. As a result, I was proudly given my own personal gym locker at the start of the season. Well, due to injuries that followed, I soon had to share my locker with an underclassman, jockstrap and all. That was a sad day.

At 16, my father sent me to an orthopedist for my persistent low back pain. After my mom and I waited over two hours with a sea of other patients, the doctor went over my x-rays. I remember crying as I saw that my spine was curved and that one of my legs was shorter than the other. His advice was to take anti-inflammatory medication, which I didn't want to do.

Later in my senior year, my dad sent me to another orthopedist for my knee injury. He was young, personable, and specialized in sports medicine.

He said I had chondromalacia patella, or runner's knee, and may need surgery. He then came back with a cortisone-filled syringe with a needle that seemed six inches long.

After seeing the look of fright on my face, he must have had a change of heart. He said, "On second thought, maybe we'll hold off on the shot for now." I was so relieved. He gave me a prescription for custom orthotics (arch supports) and anti-inflammatory medications.

The medication didn't help, so I went to be fitted for orthotics. They ended up being this rock-hard cork material and were half an inch thick. The left one was even thicker due to my shorter leg.

The orthotics were so painful in my shoes that I couldn't bear it. I brought them to college to give it another go, but they seemed impossible to walk with, never mind run with. So they became very expensive doorstops for my dorm room.

Around this time, my father (who practiced internal medicine) ran a blood test due to all my joint pain. It came back that I had elevated uric acid. He said I had gout, an inflammatory arthritis that is caused by excess uric acid crystals that deposit in the joints. He then gave me a prescription for a medication called allopurinol. I was shocked. How could I have gout when all my injuries were from sports? Well, my father had gout, so that could have a lot to do with it.

There was no internet in those days, but fortunately, there was a package insert that I read thoroughly. Not willing to risk possible kidney or liver damage and a host of other side effects, I threw the bottle away. After doing more research in the library, I changed my diet, and my uric acid levels went down to normal. I was amazed that I was able to heal my condition without medication.

That did not stop all the injuries, though. In my freshman year at Rutgers University, I joined the track team and again started having pain in both my knees. At the coach's recommendation, I went to the team's athletic trainer, who had treated a lot of knee injuries. He put an ointment on my knees, wrapped them in ACE bandages and that infamous thick white tape, and sent me on my way.

Halfway into the four-mile run back to my dorm, my knees started heating up from the pain-relieving ointment. They kept getting hotter and hotter until it felt like there were flames shooting from my knees. I abruptly stopped and tore off the bandages in the middle of the sidewalk, looking for a bucket of ice to put out the "fire."

I thought, doesn't anyone know what they're doing? How hard is it to find someone to help me with a simple knee injury, or any of my other prior injuries, for that matter?

Over the following days, my knees continued to worsen to the point that they prevented me from running at all for the first time in years. I was forced to drop off the team, and my future of competing at all seemed bleak. I was in constant pain and became very depressed, as I watched a lifelong dream of competing in the Olympics slip from my grasp.

A Change in Perspective

Something positive did evolve from all this suffering: I became deeply interested in what was causing all these illnesses and injuries. Ever since my mom brought 12-year-old me to that new health food store, I read everything I could find on nutrition and health.

My mom was into nutrition and did her best to feed us a healthy diet. But at the time, cholesterol and fat were demonized, and sugar was just fine. So, we had our regular daily dose of Ring Dings, Devil Dogs, Suzy Q's, Hostess Cupcakes, Chips Ahoy cookies, Oreos, and so on. Although soda was not allowed, except on special occasions, drinking water was not very popular, so I drank juice, Kool-Aid, juice drinks, and 1–2 quarts of milk a day.

Our Italian heritage led to plenty of pasta, bread, and cheese, and in following the popular convenience foods and health guidelines of the day, we used margarine instead of butter; soy, corn, and safflower oil instead of olive oil; and Egg Beaters instead of fresh eggs.

I also fondly remember the squirting cheese from a can, powdered milk, Carnation instant breakfast, Pop-Tarts, TV dinners, and chicken potpies. Campbell's and Lipton soup often replaced fresh, homemade soup. Of course, all this was marketed as being so healthy for you, and so convenient for the busy mom.

Unhealthy diet aside, I looked forward to when my dad would bring home the new monthly issues of medical journals for me to read: *Nutrition & the MD* and *The Physician and Sports Medicine*.

In high school, I naturally became deeply fascinated with sports injuries and how to prevent and treat them. I would read everything I could find on the subject and test things out on myself. What if I could help other kids prevent all the suffering and misery I was going through?

I decided to study exercise physiology and nutrition in college. I wanted to go into sports medicine. I didn't want to be a medical doctor after seeing what my father went through.

He said going through medical school and residency was very stressful and dehumanizing. That's where he started overeating, smoking cigarettes, and drinking gallons of coffee. He entered medical school a fit and healthy competitive swimmer. He came out an overweight chain-smoker, surviving through the endless days and nights on nothing but coffee.

As a kid, I saw him making rounds at the hospital at night, on weekends, and getting called in during the middle of the night. His health only got worse over the years. He became morbidly obese, an alcoholic, and was taking over a dozen different medications daily just to get by. It was very painful seeing this great man become gradually destroyed by his own profession.

He wasn't alone. When I visited him at the hospital, the doctors' lounge was populated by overweight doctors eating doughnuts, drinking coffee, and smoking cigarettes. It was very puzzling to me, as they were supposed to be experts in health.

In later years, I realized he was an MD: a Doctor of Medicine, not a doctor of health. That's what I chose to become: a "Doctor of Health." A doctor that specializes in getting others (and myself) healthy.

Becoming a "Doctor of Health"

In my freshman year, I decided that I could get into sports medicine by being an exercise physiologist. But, after spending two years working and doing research in the physiology lab and even having my honors thesis published in a peer-reviewed journal, I decided I was better suited to helping people directly by being a physician.

During this time, I had discovered some exercises and therapy to help my knees get better and was able to start running again. I was very encouraged that I was able to help myself when none of the medical specialists could.

Then at the start of my senior year in college, I injured my neck lifting weights. I went to many doctors, and all I received was anti-inflammatory medications and muscle relaxers. As a result, I was tired all the time, falling asleep in class, and had difficulty concentrating. My neck pain wasn't going away, and I was miserable.

When I went home at Thanksgiving, my mother, who was then divorced, brought me to her chiropractor. A chiropractor? I didn't know anything about them other than the negative comments from my college professors.

I was in so much pain, and he helped my mother, so I thought I'd give it a try. After two treatments, I dramatically improved. For the first time in two months, I could actually turn my head.

I told my chiropractor, Dr. Brian (first name), that I was very interested in sports medicine and nutrition and wanted to help others in those areas, so I was going to apply to medical schools. He said to me, "If you want to treat patients with drugs and surgery, then go to medical school. But if you want to help others get better with natural methods and without drugs and surgery, then you should consider chiropractic college. Now, you won't have the prestige of being a medical doctor, but you will be able to help a lot of patients."

I didn't know what to do at this point, so after graduating from college, I got a job at Rutgers Medical School doing research in the department of physiology. There, I got to speak to many professors and talk to students to see what they were going through. After much soul searching, I decided to apply to New York Chiropractic College, which I started the following fall.

Solving my Continued Health Problems and Sharing my Solutions

While I was in chiropractic school, my physical problems continued as I was in two car accidents. I had neck pain with numbness and tingling into my arm, and lower back pain into my left leg. Even with a lot of treatment, my pain persisted. Similarly, when I began my professional practice at age 26, I had constant stomach pain, gas, bloating, and loose stools. My abdomen hurt every day.

I continued studying nutrition extensively, trying out different things and taking numerous seminars on the latest soft tissue/muscle treatment techniques. Finally, after receiving such treatments, my pain improved considerably, but my gut issues persisted.

Unfortunately, whole-grain bread was popular at the time. I bought a bread maker and baked my own bread. However, the ingredients called for adding a packet of yeast and one teaspoon of gluten in every recipe, on top of the gluten that was already in the wheat flour. Little did I know that I was slowly killing myself.

I kept studying, going to nutrition and functional medicine seminars and using these methods on myself and patients. I did numerous tests on myself and found out I had a parasite, yeast and bacterial overgrowth in my gut.

I tried dozens of remedies to clear it up and even went to a medical doctor who gave me a prescription for two different drugs. Still no better, and each test showed the parasite was still there.

Besides the daily abdominal pain, gas, and bloating, I was tired all the time, had chronic back and joint pain, brain fog, athlete's foot, itchy ears, white spots all over my back and shoulders, and chicken skin on my arms. I also came down with prostatitis and proctalgia, which is an intermittent sudden stabbing pain in the rectum.

I ran food allergy and sensitivity testing on myself and found out I had multiple food sensitivities, including wheat, oats, legumes, yeast, and milk. I went on an elimination diet and started feeling better. After years of suffering, my stomach pain, IBS, and energy improved. I applied this knowledge with my patients and was helping a lot of people get better.

Besides continuing my education with nutrition and functional medicine, I started learning this new soft tissue treatment called Active Release Technique. I began using this extensively in my practice and got amazing results. Pretty soon I was attracting athletes from all over the state and even other countries.

One day, there was a carload of college baseball players that drove over four hours to see me. I treated each of them for their various injuries with adjustments, soft tissue treatments, and offered nutritional support. Then they drove four hours back to college the same day. They were so thrilled with the treatment results on their performance.

I remember a high school baseball player who came to see me with a nerve condition called ulnar neuropathy in his throwing arm. After all the specialists he had seen, medications, and therapy, his only recourse was "Tommy John" surgery to move the nerve to the other side of his elbow. They said this was his only option, as it was confirmed by nerve testing, and he would have permanent nerve damage and muscle wasting if the surgery was not done soon.

He was devastated, as this was the start of his senior year and would have to miss the entire season. He and his parents had been looking forward to a great season with college scholarship offers at the end.

After I treated him for four weeks with similar treatment methods, his condition cleared up and he was able to start his season on time. He was so happy and went on to play four years of college ball.

I was on top of the world. I helped so many people with their injuries and health conditions, especially young athletes. After all that I went through, it was so rewarding to be able to provide health solutions to so many whom traditional medical care had failed.

Maybe I never made it to the Olympics or set world records due to all my injuries, but I realized a greater reward was being able to help others achieve their dreams.

Developing the FreeDiet®

One Friday afternoon in July 2005, I was working at my computer when I started to experience numbness and tingling in my right hand. I received treatment after treatment, but it persisted.

I went to a neurologist, where I was given EMG and nerve conduction studies, which consisted of sending an electric current through various points on my neck and arms. It was excruciating, and I felt like I was being tortured. I found out later that the technician apparently used too much current.

The neurologist said the test confirmed I had mild carpal tunnel syndrome in my right hand. The electric current surging through my nerves caused even worse numbness and tingling in not just my right hand, but both my arms and legs.

This is crazy, I thought. How can all of this happen to me? I hoped it would go away after a few days, but it persisted relentlessly.

I continued to get treatment, including chiropractic care, muscle work, and physical therapy but was not getting better. MRIs revealed herniated discs in my neck and back. I was in constant pain and became depressed.

The numbness and tingling in my hands and feet was unrelenting. The muscles in my hands started atrophying and became very weak. It was even difficult holding my infant daughter. I was not able to exercise much at all and lost ten pounds of muscle.

I went to one doctor after another without any improvement. The neurologist recommended medications and surgery. Both of which I turned down due to the potential side effects and complications. After two years, they told me I had to stop treating patients. I was devastated.

I could not let this stop me. I hired a chiropractor to treat my patients, but I kept doing the evaluations and consulting. This allowed me to spend more time doing nutritional assessments and functional medicine.

I also poured over the research as to why this was happening to me. I read everything I could about peripheral neuropathy and nerve disorders. I did a lot more testing on myself and found some interesting things.

First, I was very deficient in vitamin D. I was shocked! I lived in Florida, the sunshine state. I went to the beach at least once a week. How was this possible? I ran other lab tests, which revealed I had hypothyroidism due to Hashimoto's thyroiditis, and rheumatoid arthritis, both of which are autoimmune diseases.

In total, I discovered I had:

- Hashimoto's
- Rheumatoid arthritis
- Vitamin D deficiency
- Low levels of vitamin B12
- Magnesium deficiency
- Blastocystis hominis, which is a parasite
- Candida/yeast and bacterial overgrowth
- High levels of mercury
- High levels of arsenic
- Adrenal fatigue/dysfunction (low cortisol levels)
- Low levels of pancreatic (digestive) enzymes
- Multiple food sensitivities, including wheat, sugar, yeast, dairy, eggs, soy, legumes, and gluten

I discovered that each of the above could contribute to the symptoms I was having. Put them all together and no wonder I had pain, fatigue, brain fog, digestive issues, and all the other problems that had plagued me over the years. This is on top of thalassemia minor (hereditary anemia), Epstein-Barr virus, MTHFR defect, and H. Pylori which I found out about later.

I had to come up with a game plan. Since I discovered that gluten sensitivity in and of itself can cause peripheral neuropathy, I would start there.

I had been eating mostly gluten free, but not 100 percent. I also still ate plenty of grains—mostly rice, millet, oats, quinoa, and corn. The gluten-free products I was eating were loaded with these, as well as yeast.

When I went completely gluten free, things improved somewhat, yet only temporarily. However, when I cut out all grains, sugar, yeast, dairy, eggs, soy, legumes, nightshades, and processed foods, I noticed a significant improvement.

This is what I now call the FreeDiet®, for one reason: because it's free of the most common food allergens that are responsible for inflammation, gut and thyroid issues, autoimmune and other chronic health conditions.

I had tried various combinations of many different nutritional supplements before, but I finally came up with a combination that worked along with this diet. I also tried dozens of parasite remedies, and I finally came across a natural parasite protocol that was effective (which I outline in Chapter 13). Over the following weeks and months, I was feeling better and better. My thyroid and rheumatoid antibodies went down to normal and have stayed that way for over ten years.

The following things improved:
- Neck and back pain cleared up
- Carpal tunnel syndrome better
- Pain and peripheral neuropathy in my arms and legs resolved
- Focus and concentration improved—the brain fog lifted
- Hashimoto's thyroiditis resolved—my antibodies decreased to normal
- Rheumatoid arthritis antibodies decreased to normal
- Abdominal pain was better
- Bloating, gas, and diarrhea cleared up
- I gained ten pounds of muscle as I was able to resume my workouts
- Rosacea and chicken skin on my arms that I had since childhood cleared up
- Athlete's foot and cracked heels gone
- Prostatitis cleared up
- Proctalgia (butt pain) resolved
- Vitamin D, vitamin B12, magnesium levels increased to normal levels
- Arsenic and mercury levels decreased to normal
- Parasite (blastocystis hominis) gone
- Candida, yeast, and bacterial overgrowth better
- Fatigue was gone and no longer depressed—I had way more energy.

The best part was that I finally started responding to the manual treatments I was receiving, and the numbness and tingling in my limbs went away. Finally, after more than three years of not being able to perform any manual therapy, I was thrilled to physically treat patients again.

I wanted to use the information I had learned to raise my practice to a whole new level. Instead of treating droves of athletes, I started seeing more and more patients with complex health issues.

Patients would come in with 20, 30, or 40 different symptoms, and they would be absolutely miserable. But I was able to help them get better. I applied the knowledge that I had learned from helping so many prior patients with the tools I had used to help myself get better against all odds.

I started seeing certain patterns repeatedly which were very similar to the health issues that I had overcome. The individualized treatment programs I would recommend also started to have similar patterns, and I have developed it over the years to get the best results.

I realized that a gluten-free diet alone doesn't work. What does work is a diet initially free of all the most common allergens, including gluten, grains, sugar, yeast, dairy, eggs, soy, legumes, nightshades, and processed foods. Of course, that is too long of a title, so what sounded great was the FreeDiet®. A diet free of inflammatory foods so you can heal your gut and thyroid and become free of pain, fatigue, fogginess, and fat.

Over the past 40 years, I have spent more than one million dollars for college, graduate school, continuing education courses, trying out over a thousand different supplements to see which works best, doing thousands of hours of research, and ordering hundreds of lab tests on myself.

I have applied this knowledge toward more than 100,000 patient visits over the last 33-plus years and interpreted thousands of lab tests, tweaking and improving my treatment protocols as I went along to help the greatest number of people. I have done all this work so you don't have to.

I am constantly applying the health principles in this book to my own life, as I, too, would like to stay looking and feeling young and enjoying vibrant health. I see myself as a role model for others, to give them hope, to show them that, yes, it can be done. You can get better.

Through reading this FreeDiet® book, you can take advantage of all the knowledge I've used to help myself and thousands of patients, and you can apply it to your own life. If you do, I believe you will start to be free of your pain and chronic health conditions, heal your gut and thyroid, and live a healthy, free, and vibrant life.

CHAPTER 2

THE FREEDIET® MINDSET: WHAT IS YOUR WHY?

Before you get started on the FreeDiet® itself, let's dive into why you are doing this. In other words, what would you like to see as a result?

Check off your health goals below in the initial column, and you will be able to track your improvement as you go through the program. Listed are the most common health goals for my patients, and you can write any others you have at the bottom.

Then take the Health Assessment Quiz to see where you are. I do this with each of my patients at the beginning of care to get a baseline and measure their progress. You can repeat this again after 28 days on FreeDiet® Phase 1 so you can see all the improvements, and then again after a month on Phase 2.

My health goals include:

Health Goals	Initial Check off	Phase 1 % better	Phase 2 % better
Date:			
Have more energy			
Digestive symptoms (i.e. constipation, diarrhea, gas, bloating, indigestion) cleared up			
Become pain free			
Concentration and memory improved—brain fog resolved			
Anxiety and/or depression better			
Sleep better			
Headaches resolved			

Vertigo/dizziness better			
Sinuses clear			
Thyroid improvement			
Skin improved			
Hair loss better			
Blood pressure and/or cholesterol normalized			
Hormones balanced			
Achieve my ideal weight of ___ lbs./kg			
Other:			

HEALTH ASSESSMENT QUIZ

Enter the following score on each line:

0 for rarely or never have symptom

1 for mild or occasionally have

2 for moderate or sometimes have

3 for severe or frequently have

Symptom/condition	Initial	Phase 1	Phase 2
Date:			
Fatigue/tired/sluggish			
Brain fog (lack of focus and concentration)			
Poor memory			
Headaches/migraines			
Dizziness/vertigo			
Faintness/unsteadiness/lack of balance			
Tremors			
Insomnia			
Anxiety			
Depression			
Anger or irritability			
Mood swings			
Sinus congestion and/or postnasal drip			

Tinnitus (ear ringing/noises)			
Itchy ears			
Ears clogged or aching			
Watery or itchy eyes			
Swollen or sticky eyelids			
Puffiness or dark circles under eyes			
Indigestion			
Heartburn			
Reflux			
Difficulty swallowing or lump in throat			
Abdominal pain			
Nausea			
Vomiting			
Abdominal bloating			
Belching			
Gas			
Bad breath			
Constipation			
Diarrhea			
Rectal itching			
Heart palpitations			
Rapid heartbeat			
High blood pressure			
Cold hands and/or feet			
Leg cramps or twitching at night			
Chest congestion or wheezing			
Chest pain			
Asthma			
Difficulty breathing			
Shortness of breath			
Chronic cough			
Sore throat			
Swollen tongue/gums/lips			
White coating on tongue			
Canker sores			
Acne			
Rashes or hives			

Itchy skin			
Dry skin			
Eczema or psoriasis			
Nail fungus			
Cracked heels or soles of feet			
Dry, flaking scalp			
Sensitive to smells and chemicals			
Hair loss or thinning			
Hot flashes or excessive perspiration			
PMS symptoms			
Menstrual cramps			
Frequently getting sick			
Repeated urinary tract infections			
Genital itch or discharge			
Overweight/difficulty losing weight			
Water retention/overall bloating			
Underweight/difficulty gaining weight			
Neck, back, or joint pain			
TMJ/jaw pain			
Muscle aches/pains/stiffness			
Arthritis			
Numbness or tingling			
Stinging, burning, or electric shock sensations			
Other:			
Total Score:			

A 0-5 total score with no individual scores of 2 or 3

B 5-10 total score with less than two individual scores of 2 or 3

C 10-20 total score with less than four individual scores of 2 or 3

D 20-30 total score with less than five individual scores of 2 or 3

F >30 total score with five or more individual scores of 2 or 3

How did you score? How about you add another goal to reduce your score by 50 percent after 28 days on the FreeDiet®? How about going from being a D student to B, an F to a C, or even better in the first semester?

Once you have your goals and your why, it will be easier to stick with the program, especially as you're faced with that loaf of bread, ice cream, or double chocolate cake.

For me, as I was becoming free of all my symptoms, I realized that eating certain foods was not worth the consequences. People may say to me that I am missing out on the finer things in life and depriving myself, but I know how much better I feel when I eat like this, and I simply don't want to go back to how it was before. Not even for a day.

I also don't want to end up like my father. I saw the pain and misery he went through. By inadvertently violating every rule of the FreeDiet®, he was in pain, morbidly obese, had arthritis, diabetes, heart disease, and depression, and had to take a dozen medications just to get through the day. I certainly want to avoid that.

I see the body as a sacred temple. I was given this gift, and I need to take care of it. I take care of my car by using premium gas, getting regular oil changes and wheel alignments, paying for tune-ups, and so on. I wash and detail the car and keep the tires inflated to the proper pressure for a smooth ride.

I do all this, and yet we typically keep our automobile for three to nine years. We keep our bodies 80-plus years. Shouldn't we give our bodies at least the same level of care as we do our vehicles?

I had a 60-year-old patient named Robert who followed the FreeDiet® and was doing great. He lost 28 pounds, his gallbladder and digestive issues were better, his chronic knee pain cleared up, and he was able to exercise for the first time in months.

Then he decided to go to a pancake breakfast, and he ended up with a gallbladder attack, which he had been free of since starting the program. Listen, if you have a gluten sensitivity and feel great avoiding gluten, grains, sugar, and yeast, you can't suddenly eat a pile of pancakes without repercussions. It's not a good idea to have a cheat day on the FreeDiet®, especially in Phase 1.

So many parents diligently take care of their kids, driving them all over town. Their kids join travel teams and suddenly parents are driving them all over the state, sometimes driving eight or more hours in one weekend to sit on metal bleachers for hours on end.

There is no time for yourself, so you get out of shape and start having anxiety, fatigue, and insomnia. Your relationship with your spouse suffers. You go to bed too late because there is so much to do. Your kids are well taken care of. Meanwhile, you feel miserable inside.

You have to first decide what's important to you. Ask yourself:
- Is my health important to me?
- Do I want my life back?
- Do I want to feel good again?
- What do I want to see happen in the next few months?
- How do I want to look and feel?
- How do I set up a routine so I can reach my goals?

Write out the answers to these questions. If you said yes to any of the above, it's time to start scheduling exercise, healthy meals, and a morning ritual to start the day off right.

When I was growing up, my parents let us six kids do a lot on our own. We did not get rides all over town for playdates, no rides to school, no rides to practice or games. We made our own breakfast and packed our own lunch for school. At age 12, I was even cooking dinner for all eight of us after my mother broke her leg.

Things are a little different today. I know one mom who drives her daughter 90 minutes to swim team practice in the morning before school. She then waits for her during practice and drives her home. After school, she drives her back down, watches her practice, and drives her back home. Meanwhile, her own health is suffering.

What about you? Ask yourself the following additional questions:
1. How can I be my best self?
2. What do I need to start doing to feel great?
3. What do I need to stop doing?
4. How do I need to set up my schedule so that I can exercise and take care of myself?

Do you want to look attractive and feel desirable as you get older? You can retain that vibrancy of your youth, be energetic and full of life, attractive and in shape; instead of feeling worn out and exhausted and letting yourself go. We all want to look good, feel good, be alert and full of energy.

It all comes down to your belief system and routine. You don't need to struggle with making good choices daily. You don't need the intense discipline to avoid all the addictive, unhealthy, sugary junk foods. All you have to do is ask yourself the right questions and decide to turn your health and your life around. Decide to be free of pain, fatigue, fogginess, fat, and misery. Develop the thinking and belief system to get and keep yourself healthy and feeling great. You can do this with the FreeDiet®.

When I was a child, growing up Catholic, we were not allowed to eat meat on Fridays. It was not hard to do that because it was just the rule. It required no discipline. That was our belief system. It was routine. Every Friday we had fish or pasta or something other than meat.

Orthodox Jews choose to only eat kosher food. They do not have to think about it. It's a belief system, a routine; it's automatic. Cows are roaming the streets in India without fear of being slaughtered for a hamburger. The locals do not have to give much thought to not eating beef. It's just part of their belief system, their daily routine. It's automatic.

In the same way, my belief is that my body is sacred, and I consume only foods that are going to allow me to feel good and stay healthy. I don't want to go back and feel the pain and misery, the digestive and skin problems, the neuropathy and the fatigue that I had before.

That's my vision for you. That you get to the place that you are not going to put up with the misery anymore. That you make a commitment to stick with this and achieve vibrant health.

Again, decide that you want to feel amazing and ask yourself:
- Is my health important to me?
- Do I want my life back?
- Do I want to feel good again?
- Do I want to look and feel younger?
- Am I willing to carve out time for myself and set up a routine so I can reach my goals?
- Am I committed to seeing this happen over the next three months?

If so, then read the next chapter to start the FreeDiet® Phase 1. You absolutely can reach your goals. You can be *free* again and feel the best you have in years!

CHAPTER 3

THE FREEDIET® PHASE 1

The FreeDiet® Phase 1 is *free* of foods most commonly responsible for inflammation, as well as digestive, thyroid, and other chronic health issues, including weight loss resistance. This is where you can really start to notice the improved energy, mental clarity, weight loss, and a reduction of pain and many other chronic symptoms. Again, you can become *free* of pain, fatigue, brain fog, and excess fat. You can start to look and feel younger and more vibrant.

The FreeDiet® Phase 1 is *free* of gluten, grains, sugar, yeast, dairy, eggs, soy, legumes, nightshades, and processed foods.

Essentially what you CAN eat during this phase are proteins, vegetables, fruit, and essential fats. Refer to the FreeDiet® Phase 1 chart in this chapter for over 80 foods that are allowed. The following is a summary of what that looks like daily.

Breakfast

The ideal breakfast during Phase 1 and Phase 2 is a protein smoothie. I call this the FreeDiet® 3-Minute Super Smoothie. It's fast, easy, and a great way to start your day. Since you're avoiding eggs, grains, and dairy, this is the best option for a fulfilling breakfast. It's a great source of protein, fruits and vegetables, healthy fats, and fiber. It's very nourishing, very cleansing, and it only takes three minutes to make.

The FreeDiet® 3-Minute Super Smoothie

You will need:

- 12 oz. water
- ½ cup frozen organic blueberries or cherries
- 1 serving FreeDiet™ Protein, Paleo Protein, or Organic Pea Protein
- 1 scoop FreeGreens™ Organic Superfood Powder
- 1 Tbsp. ground flaxseeds
- 1 tsp. Organic Psyllium Husk Powder, gradually increasing to 1 Tbsp. over 1–2 weeks
- 1 Tbsp. organic unrefined coconut oil
- 1 blender to mix ingredients

Blend the water and organic blueberries or cherries for 5 seconds.

Then add the protein, FreeGreens™, ground flaxseeds, psyllium, and coconut oil, and blend for another 5 seconds.

Drink and enjoy within a few minutes, as it can get very thick with the fiber. At any time, add more water if too thick.

This is a great solution to a healthy breakfast for the following reasons:

The blueberries and cherries are very high in polyphenols and antioxidants, which can support healthy brain function and inflammatory response.

Unrefined coconut oil is a healthy source of essential fats and medium-chain triglycerides (MCT), which are fuel for the brain.

FreeDiet™ Protein and Paleo Protein are from a purified beef protein containing both complete and collagen proteins that are naturally found in beef. It is sourced from animals raised in Sweden without hormones or GMOs. It has a significant amount of collagen from bone broth, so besides muscle support, it also can support healthy cartilage, ligaments, hair, skin, nails, and gut permeability—great for leaky gut.

The Organic Pea Protein is an excellent source of plant-based amino acids, which are the building blocks of the body, and is high in iron. Pea protein has a very low allergy potential and is easily digestible.

FreeGreens™ Organic Superfood Powder is a proprietary formula that includes organic ingredients with the optimal balance of greens, vegetables, fruits, herbs, and plant sources to provide premium natural sources of nutrients, antioxidants, liver and digestive support, fiber, blood glucose balance, and healthy inflammatory response.

Ground flaxseeds are an excellent source of omega-3s, fiber, and plant lignans.

Organic Psyllium Husk Powder is a soluble fiber that helps keep you regular and is very cleansing for the intestines. That, combined with the coconut oil, makes this very filling and feels like a complete breakfast.

Note:

If you add everything at once and blend, it can get too thick with the psyllium. The same goes if you over blend. Simply follow the instructions above for the best results.

For a more filling meal as well as some crunch, you can add dehydrated coconut chips and/or soaked nuts at the end and blend for a few seconds.

For nut milk instead of water, use a handful of soaked nuts (especially cashews) or coconut chunks and add to 12 oz. water initially. Blend well before adding the fruit and powders.

At any time if the smoothie is too thick, add more water.

The 3-Minute Super Smoothie is an important part of the FreeDiet® since it's a great source of protein, fruits and vegetables, healthy fats, and fiber. It's both very nourishing and very cleansing. If you're in an area where you don't have the ingredients available to you and are unable to make a smoothie, a less preferable option is to have leftovers from dinner or have soaked raw nuts and coconut with berries.

Lunch and Dinner

Lunch and dinner are quite simple. Proteins, vegetables, and essential fats.

Choose from one of the following proteins: fish, chicken, turkey, beef, lamb (approximately four ounces) with plenty of vegetables and/or salad. For your vegetables and salad, you can use extra virgin olive oil and lemon, lime, salt, or one of the other amazing dressings from Chapter 19.

The best protein choices are organic grass-fed beef, organic chicken, and wild salmon. If you are a vegan, you can choose soaked nuts and/or seeds for your protein.

Dinner should be finished at least three hours before bedtime. If you are in bed by 10 PM, finish by 7 PM. This should give you approximately 12 hours before eating breakfast if you eat at 7 AM the next morning.

Snacks

For the best results. I recommend only three meals a day—breakfast, lunch, and dinner. Some people do better with snacking, like those with hypoglycemia or those who are underweight. If you need to snack, choose from the following:

Midmorning or afternoon snacks:
- The FreeDiet® 3-Minute Super Smoothie
- FreeGreens™ Organic Superfood Powder
- Raw vegetables with homemade dressings/dips. See Chapter 19 for recipes.
- Raw walnuts, pecans, cashews, hazelnuts, Brazil or macadamia nuts, preferably organic.

Before eating, make sure you soak them. See below for why and how to soak nuts. You can also refer to this video at nmcwellness.com/how-and-why-to-soak-nuts.

Why should you soak nuts (and seeds) before eating?
1. Most nuts are covered with fungus—mold and yeast.
2. Most nuts are fumigated with pesticides unless they are organic.
3. Nuts are high in lectins, oxalates, phytic acids, and enzyme inhibitors, which can interfere with nutrient absorption and cause other digestive issues.

Soaking helps with all the above. Soaking makes them more digestible, less bitter and improves their taste. While someone with a true nut allergy should still avoid them, I found that many sensitivity reactions people have with nuts, as in autoimmune, skin, and digestive conditions, are avoided by properly soaking them.

How to Soak Nuts
Place raw nuts into a glass jar or bowl.
Cover with filtered water, by at least ½ inch over the top of nuts (because they expand).
Add 1 Tbsp. of salt per quart of water as an option.
Leave on the counter for 12–24 hours.

You can then change the water and place it in the refrigerator, where you can keep nuts for up to five days if you change the water daily.

For nut milk and recipes, you can use the soaked nuts without dehydrating or roasting. Otherwise, they taste better if you do the following.

To dry the nuts:

You can sprinkle some salt over the nuts beforehand. For pecans, cinnamon with monk fruit or stevia powder tastes great.

If you have a dehydrator, spread them out on the trays and dehydrate at 120 degrees Fahrenheit for 24 to 48 hours, until crisp. See the Resources section in the back of this book for a dehydrator recommendation.

Or place in your oven at the typical lowest setting, which is 175–200 degrees Fahrenheit. Depending on the temperature you choose and the type of nut, bake/roast for 4–10 hours or until crisp. You can use a higher temperature if you want them done faster.

Other FreeDiet® tips:

Since you're avoiding canned, processed, and packaged foods, you will be getting much less sodium than usual. I generally recommend using 1 teaspoon of sea salt or Himalayan salt for your total daily intake.

Drink plenty of filtered water throughout the day, especially between meals. You can squeeze fresh lemon or lime in your water or some FreeGreens™ Organic Superfood Powder. Also, see the flavored water recipes in Chapter 19.

A general recommendation is to drink half of your body weight in ounces. For example, a 160-pound person will drink 80 ounces (10 cups or approximately 2.5 liters) of water. Drink more if engaging in outdoor activities or exercise that causes you to perspire.

If you want to avoid getting up to urinate at night, drink most of your water earlier in the day and afternoon so you can keep your water consumption in the evening to a minimum.

Filtered water is best, and the water purifiers I recommend are in the resource section at the back of the book.

This chart offers a detailed description of the allowed foods and the foods to avoid during the FreeDiet® Phase 1.

Food Groups	Allowed	Avoid
Proteins	Chicken and turkey (except ground), lamb, beef, bison, fish (salmon, sole, sardines, flounder, pollock, Atlantic cod, Atlantic mackerel) Best choices: organic poultry, grass-fed beef and lamb, wild-caught fish	Barbecued or blackened meats, cold cuts, ham, pork, hot dogs, sausage, ground chicken, ground turkey, smoked or canned meats and fish, eggs, shrimp and shellfish, bluefish, grouper, halibut, king mackerel, mahi-mahi, marlin, orange roughy, shark, swordfish, tilefish, tuna, sea bass, tilapia, imitation crab
Legumes	None (except pea protein)	All beans, peas, green beans, lentils, soybeans, tofu, miso, tempeh, alfalfa
Dairy	Organic Ghee (clarified butter)	Cow and goat milk, cheese, yogurt, kefir, cottage cheese, cream, butter, ice cream, non-dairy creamers
Starch/ Grains	Squash (i.e. butternut, acorn, spaghetti squash), cauliflower rice	Gluten: wheat, rye, barley, couscous, malt, spelt, Kamut, oats, corn, rice, amaranth, tapioca, buckwheat, arrowroot, millet, quinoa, sorghum, teff, pasta, bread, toast, cookies, cakes, chips, crackers, popcorn, white potato, sweet and Hannah potato, yams, yuca (cassava)
Vegetables	Fresh or frozen (preferably organic): romaine lettuce, arugula, butter lettuce, cucumber, avocado, radishes, celery, fennel, asparagus, artichoke, watercress, jicama Cooked: kale, collards, cabbage, broccoli, cauliflower, bok choy, Brussels sprouts, turnips, turnip greens, garlic, onion, chayote squash, rutabaga, organic yellow squash and zucchini	Corn, mushrooms, eggplant, white potatoes, peppers, tomatoes, carrots, parsnips, sunchokes, beets, rhubarb, beet greens, callaloo, Swiss chard, spinach, green beans, all canned or creamed vegetables Raw: kale, collards, cabbage, broccoli, cauliflower, bok choy, Brussels sprouts
Soups	Homemade soups with no bullion	Bullion, canned or boxed soups, cream soups

Food Groups	Allowed	Avoid
Fruits	Fresh and frozen fruit with no added sugar (preferably organic): blueberries, cherries, cranberries, lemon, lime, apricot, coconut, kiwi, peach, pear, plum, organic papaya, pomegranate, starfruit, small or 1/2 apple *Up to 1 serving/cup per day*	Orange, grapefruit, tangerine, mandarin orange, blackberries, raspberries, strawberries; dried fruit, such as raisins, figs, and dates; canned fruits, ackee, banana, breadfruit, jackfruit, goji berry, soursop, mango, pineapple, plantain, grapes, cantaloupe, honeydew, watermelon
Fats/Oils, Nuts, and Seeds	Cold/expeller-pressed, unrefined, extra virgin olive and coconut oil, avocado oil; ground flaxseeds, hemp seeds Raw, soaked: walnuts, cashews, pecans, hazelnuts, macadamia nuts, Brazil nuts, pine nuts, chestnuts, pumpkin seeds, tiger nuts	Margarine, shortening, refined oils, soy, corn and canola oil, mayonnaise, salad dressings, peanuts, pistachios, almonds, chia, sunflower and sesame seeds, nut butter
Beverages	Filtered water, non-citrus herbal tea (gluten-free), green tea (organic), homemade nut and coconut milk	Milk: cow, goat, soy, rice, almond; fruit juice and drinks, coffee, black tea, cocoa, alcohol, beer, wine, Champagne, soda, sports drinks, coconut water, seltzer, kefir, kombucha
Sweeteners	Stevia, monk fruit (lo han guo)	High fructose corn syrup, corn syrup, agave, rice syrup, white or brown sugar, cane sugar, dehydrated cane juice, malt, fruit juice concentrate, honey, molasses, dextrose, glucose, maple syrup, coconut sugar and nectar, erythritol, xylitol (non-GMO birch), aspartame, acesulfame K, saccharin, sucralose
Spices and condiments	Himalayan or sea salt, gluten-free herbs and spices, including basil, chives, cilantro, cinnamon, cloves, coriander, cumin, dill weed, garlic, ginger, lemongrass, mace, onion powder, oregano, parsley, peppermint, rosemary, saffron, sage, spearmint, thyme, turmeric, vanilla	Black or white pepper, cayenne, chili pepper, curry, nutmeg, paprika, red pepper, vinegar (all including apple cider vinegar), salsa, ketchup, mustard, mayonnaise, relish, barbecue and steak sauce, soy and teriyaki sauce, miso, tempeh, tofu, coconut aminos, canned foods, olives, pickled and fermented foods, chocolate/cacao, yeast-containing products, nutritional and brewer's yeast (saccharomyces cerevisiae)

Frequently asked questions — Why should I avoid...?

Ground chicken and turkey

Store bought ground chicken and turkey contain flavor enhancers that either have gluten or yeast extracts. I've had three patients in a span of two months have negative reactions to ground turkey. This was three different brands, and one of them was organic and gluten free.

The first patient was a 24-year-old woman who is highly gluten sensitive, with celiac markers. She called me up because she was breaking out in hives all over her body and her lips had swelled up. She ended up at the urgent care center and needed some medication for the allergic response.

I asked her if she was eating anything different that may have contained gluten or yeast. She said no, as she was only eating foods that were in the FreeDiet® Phase 1.

I said, "Well, you have any changed anything recently? What are you eating for breakfast, lunch, and dinner?"

She said, "Oh, well, over the last two weeks I started using ground turkey instead of ground beef because I thought it was healthier."

The brand was gluten free and she still had that reaction. She does fine with eating regular chicken or turkey, however. Within two days of cutting out the ground meat, her skin rash and swelling cleared up, and she was back to feeling good again.

The next two patients had digestive symptoms that already cleared up on the FreeDiet® Phase 1 but had come back when they started eating ground turkey. Third time's a charm. I decided to add it to the "*avoid*" foods column.

If you have a meat grinder at home, however, you can certainly make and consume your own ground turkey or chicken. This way you can use your own approved spices and make sure it's FreeDiet® friendly.

Eggplant, white potatoes, peppers, tomatoes

These are called nightshades, which is a family of plants that also includes chili powder, cayenne pepper, curry, paprika, and goji berries. Some people, especially those with autoimmune conditions or leaky gut, can have an inflammatory reaction to these.

Sweet potatoes, parsnips, yuca, beets

Although these can be very healthy for you, we are avoiding most starchy vegetables in the FreeDiet® Phase 1 because of their higher carbohydrate and/or sugar content.

Raw: kale, collards, cabbage, broccoli, cauliflower, bok choy, Brussels sprouts

These are more difficult to digest unless cooked.

Carrots

Carrots are higher in sugar than most vegetables. Even though they are healthy for you, in the FreeDiet® Phase 1, we are keeping sugar intake to a minimum.

Certain Fruits

Fruits that are more commonly allergenic, have higher sugar content, or have a propensity to have yeast/mold on them, like strawberries, are avoided.

Almonds

Based on my personal experience and on lab tests of numerous patients, almonds are the nuts that are most commonly reactive. They are also the nuts highest in oxalates.

Apple Cider Vinegar, Kombucha, and Kefir

Due to the yeast content of all three, and high sugar content in many types of kombucha and kefir, these are to be avoided. I understand that there are health benefits to these, but we are avoiding sugar and yeast in the early phases of the FreeDiet®.

Most of the patients I see with chronic health conditions have yeast overgrowth and/or sensitivity. I've seen countless patients with itchy skin, dandruff, frequent urinary tract and yeast infections, brain fog, moodiness, itchy ears, sticky eyelids, and sinus congestion all become aggravated by consuming the above three foods.

When I was dealing with IBS and Candida, whenever I would eat foods that contained gluten, yeast, or sugar, I would have abdominal bloating and my ears started itching. This happened with bread, wine, kombucha, kefir, and even apple cider vinegar. Even though the latter three were supposed to be beneficial for yeast overgrowth.

Do I have to eat organic foods?

I recommend consuming organic foods whenever possible, based on availability and your budget. This includes fruits, vegetables, nuts, and seeds. Another option is to buy organic for at least the produce with the highest pesticide residues. The list below is Environmental Working Group's 12 foods with the highest pesticide content.

EWG'S DIRTY DOZEN FOR 2019

Strawberries	Peaches
Spinach	Cherries
Kale	Pears
Nectarines	Tomatoes
Apples	Celery
Grapes	Potatoes

For a PDF version of the FreeDiet® Phase 1 food chart and shopping list, see the Free Gift section at the front of the book.

The FreeDiet® Phase 1 Shopping List

Proteins
- Beef, grass-fed
- Bison, grass-fed
- Lamb, grass-fed
- Chicken, preferably organic (not ground)
- Turkey, preferably organic (not ground)
- Fish: wild salmon, sole, flounder, sardines, pollock, Atlantic cod, Atlantic mackerel

Vegetables (preferably organic)
- Artichoke
- Arugula
- Avocado (fruit)
- Butter lettuce
- Celery
- Cucumbers
- Fennel
- Jicama
- Radishes
- Romaine lettuce
- Watercress

For cooking:
- Acorn squash
- Asparagus
- Bok choy
- Broccoli
- Brussels sprouts
- Butternut squash
- Cabbage
- Cauliflower
- Chayote squash
- Collards
- Garlic
- Kale
- Onion
- Rutabaga
- Spaghetti squash
- Starfruit
- Turnips
- Turnip greens
- Yellow squash, organic
- Zucchini, organic

Fruits (preferably organic)

- Apple
- Apricot
- Blueberries
- Cherries
- Coconut
- Kiwi
- Lemon
- Lime
- Papaya, organic
- Peach
- Pear
- Plum
- Pomegranate
- Starfruit

Oils (cold/expeller-pressed, unrefined, extra virgin, preferably organic)

- Avocado oil
- Coconut oil
- Ghee (clarified butter)
- Olive oil

Nuts/Seeds (preferably raw and organic)

- Brazil nuts
- Cashews
- Chestnuts
- Hemp seeds
- Flaxseeds
  (for grinding at home) or
- Ground flaxseeds
- Hazelnuts
- Macadamia nuts
- Pecans
- Pine nuts
- Pumpkin seeds
- Tiger nuts
- Walnuts

Beverages

- Filtered water
- Green tea, organic
- Herbal tea, non-citrus (gluten-free)

Sweeteners

- Stevia
- Monk fruit (lo han guo)

Spices (preferably organic)

- Basil
- Chives
- Cilantro
- Cinnamon
- Cloves
- Coriander
- Cumin
- Dill weed
- Garlic
- Ginger
- Himalayan or sea salt
- Lemongrass
- Mace
- Mint
- Onion powder
- Oregano
- Parsley
- Peppermint
- Rosemary
- Saffron
- Sage
- Spearmint
- Thyme
- Turmeric
- Vanilla (not vanillin)

Frozen Foods (preferably organic)

- Blueberries
- Cherries
- Artichokes
- Asparagus
- Broccoli
- Brussels sprouts
- Cauliflower
- Cauliflower rice
- Collards
- Kale

The FreeDiet® 14-Day Sample Meal Plan

This is a sample meal plan with included recipes from Chapter 19.

You can use this in one of three ways:

1. Follow this plan if you like to create delicious new recipes each day.
2. Use this as a guideline. For instance, on Day 2 Dinner, replace salmon and artichokes with any other allowed fish and vegetables. Then you can try one of the new recipes as time permits when you want to be creative.
3. Follow the FreeDiet® general guidelines—FreeDiet® 3-minute super smoothie for breakfast; protein, vegetables, and healthy fat for lunch and dinner.

	Breakfast	Lunch	Dinner
Day 1	FreeDiet® 3-minute super smoothie	Healing Chicken Soup	Healing Chicken Soup
Day 2	FreeDiet® 3-minute super smoothie	Healing Chicken Soup	Artichoke Encrusted Salmon Cauliflower Rice
Day 3	FreeDiet® 3-minute super smoothie	Leftovers with salad*	Easy Meatloaf Broccoli
Day 4	FreeDiet® 3-minute super smoothie	Leftovers with salad	Thai Cauliflower Soup Zucchini Cakes
Day 5	FreeDiet® 3-minute super smoothie	Leftovers with salad	Citrus Crusted Cod Brussels Sprouts
Day 6	FreeDiet® 3-minute super smoothie	Leftovers with salad	Basil and Artichoke Stuffed Chicken with Cashew Cheese Spaghetti Squash
Day 7	FreeDiet® 3-minute super smoothie	Leftovers with salad	Steak Fajitas Asparagus
Day 8	FreeDiet® 3-minute super smoothie	Leftovers with salad	Creamy Butternut Soup
Day 9	FreeDiet® 3-minute super smoothie	Leftovers with salad	Salmon Cakes Bok choy
Day 10	FreeDiet® 3-minute super smoothie	Leftovers with salad	Coconut Crusted Chicken with Sweet Lime Sauce Broccoli

Day 11	FreeDiet® 3-minute super smoothie	Leftovers with salad	Paleo Meatballs Zucchini Noodles with Creamy Cashew Sauce
Day 12	FreeDiet® 3-minute super smoothie	Leftovers with salad	Hazelnut Encrusted Flounder Asparagus
Day 13	FreeDiet® 3-minute super smoothie	Leftovers with salad	Avocado Curry Chicken Salad Cauliflower Rice
Day 14	FreeDiet® 3-minute super smoothie	Leftovers with salad	Cauliflower Cakes Brussels Sprouts

*Salad

Start with romaine lettuce, butter lettuce, and/or arugula and add celery, cucumber, fennel, radish, and watercress to your liking. Avocados are also an excellent addition to your salad and are full of healthy fat.

Salad Dressings

Choose between:

Extra virgin olive oil and lemon or lime

Extra virgin olive oil with Himalayan or sea salt

Or Refer to Chapter 19:

Zesty Lemon Dressing

Creamy Chive and Garlic Dressing

Ranch-O-Yum Dressing

The FreeDiet® Progress Chart

Track your progress from day 1.

Name:			Height:	
Week	Date	Weight	Waist (inches or cm)	Blood Pressure
0 (Start)				
1				
2				
3				
4				
5				
6				
7				
8				
9				
10				
11				
12				
13				
14				
15				

Keep in mind...

If it seems overwhelming that there is nothing to eat, and all your foods were taken away from you, that's actually a good thing. Many of those foods were probably the same ones making you feel miserable! Remember, there are over 80 foods in the allowed list in the FreeDiet® Phase 1. Once you establish routines and start feeling better, it can become quite easy to follow.

In the next chapter, I will review overcoming challenges and how to stick with FreeDiet® and succeed.

CHAPTER 4

OVERCOMING CHALLENGES— HOW TO STICK WITH THE FREEDIET® AND SUCCEED

After working with thousands of patients on the FreeDiet®, one of the biggest measures of success is getting through that first week. Especially in those first few days, there are withdrawal symptoms from gluten, sugar, and any other foods you may be sensitive to, with symptoms like headaches, irritability, moodiness, and fatigue. I had one five-year-old patient that, according to his mom, was on the floor kicking and screaming, which is how a lot of us feel inside without our fix.

The key to getting through this is to know that it is temporary. This too shall pass. Know that as you get through the first week—especially the first three or four days—you will start to feel a whole lot better. Almost everyone tells me that by the beginning of the second week they have more energy, less brain fog, clearer thinking, improved digestive symptoms, better sleep, and fewer aches and pains. Plus, if they need to lose weight, it usually starts dropping easily by this time.

It's very important to keep following the plan 100 percent, no matter how hard the first few days become. Keep the reason why you're doing this at the forefront of your mind and see yourself getting there. Remember, no "good" food is worth feeling bad.

Having a support system really helps also. A 35-year-old patient named Juan was going through his first week of the FreeDiet® with major withdrawal symptoms, mainly from coffee, gluten, and sugar. He was miserable, tired, depressed, frustrated, hungry, and was having constant headaches. He wanted to quit, but his wife kept encouraging him. He got through it, and his headaches resolved, his constipation, gas, and bloating cleared up, he had a better overall mood, his insomnia improved, and his chronic joint pain was much better. He also dropped ten pounds in the first two weeks!

What about cheat days?

What about cheat days with your spouse? Do you say, "Well, honey, I'm loyal to you six days a week, but Sunday's my cheat day. It's just one day. Is that okay? That's not a problem, is it?"

Can you imagine your kid telling you, "But Mom, I only cheat on my tests once in a while. It's really not that big of a deal. Most of the time I don't cheat."

It's the same thing with the FreeDiet®. Once you start cheating, guilt floods you, and those cravings come back—and it doesn't end there. That one, itty-bitty cheat day affects every other day.

Be consistent and stay true to yourself. There is a time for reintroducing foods in FreeDiet® Phase 2 and beyond, but there's a system to it that allows you to maintain the improvements you'll experience in the FreeDiet® Phase 1.

Cheat days don't work with the FreeDiet®. Eating a food you have a sensitivity to can raise your antibodies for three weeks, so even occasional cheating means you're not allowing the inflammation to calm down. Your body needs a chance to heal, and cheat days prevent that. Cheat days can also increase your cravings and make it more difficult to stick with the program and get the results you're looking for.

Juan cheated with one just cookie in week two of the FreeDiet®. He thought it was no big deal because he used to eat them all the time. The next morning, he woke up with diarrhea and joint pain in both hands that had previously cleared up. No more cheating for him.

A 62-year-old patient named Steven was doing great on the FreeDiet®. In the first 28 days, he lost 22 pounds, his life-long digestive symptoms had improved, chronic pain resolved, fatigue and insomnia were better, blood pressure decreased 30 points to normal, and he was able to drop many of his medications.

He felt so good that at a certain point he started cheating occasionally, with things like chips, bread, or a chicken sandwich. As his cravings increased, he began cheating more regularly. He quickly gained ten pounds, his diarrhea, gas, abdominal pain, and bloating returned, and his blood pressure became high again.

Stick with what works and stay the course! You can do this and get the results you're looking for!

How can I do this if I don't have enough time and I'm just too busy?

Breakfast takes less than five minutes, cleanup and all, so you do have time for that. See the FreeDiet® 3-Minute Super Smoothie in Chapter 19 recipes and watch the video at nmcwellness.com/dr-toms-3-minute-super-smoothie-recipe.

The easiest thing for lunch is leftovers from dinner. Let's say you make chicken and vegetables with a salad for dinner, which may only take 30 minutes. Make enough so you have leftovers, which you put in a glass storage container in the fridge. The next day, have that for lunch.

You could even make enough leftovers to get a second dinner and lunch the day after that. Add some variety by using the dressings in Chapter 19. For example, by making chicken or salmon salad for lunch.

At home, we use a countertop steam convection oven that has saved us a lot of time. You could take frozen wild salmon with some frozen vegetables, put it on steam bake at 275 degrees, and it's done in about 20 minutes.

My wife also likes the Instant Pot cooker which makes cooking an entire meal simple and quick. See the Resources in the back section of this book for the steam oven and Instant Pot we use and recommend.

If you would rather not cook at all, then there are several healthy meal services that can make and deliver all your meals. They can accommodate your needs and make all your FreeDiet®-compliant meals for you. You have your FreeDiet® 3-Minute Super Smoothie for breakfast, and they'll do the rest. Problem solved!

How am I going to make my own meals when I also have to cook for my children and my spouse?

One solution to do this is to start making the new recipes in Chapter 19. You don't have to announce to everyone that you're on this special diet that is free of gluten, grains, sugar, yeast, dairy, eggs, soy, legumes, nightshades, and processed foods. You also don't have to announce that everyone in the family must eat like this. Once you start making some of the new, delicious recipes, your kids and spouse will often ask you to make it again—without even realizing how healthy it is.

Sometimes the differences are small. Maybe the only difference between your family's steak dinner and your own is that they're eating potatoes, rice, or pasta as a side dish and you're not. Or, you can make the cauliflower rice recipe instead of regular rice and not even tell them ahead of time. With the proper seasonings, they may not know the difference. As for eating pasta, you can substitute grain-free pasta for them and not even tell until after they say they like it. The sauce can make all the difference. See Chapter 19 for an amazing pesto sauce and other recipes.

Well, everyone in my house and my friends are eating things around me that I'm not supposed to eat.

Yes, you're going to have challenges and temptations. Ask yourself: Is it worth it? Remember why you are doing the FreeDiet® and what your goals are. Do you want to be free of chronic pain, headaches, digestive issues, fatigue, brain fog, skin problems, and improve your thyroid? Do you want to finally get down to your ideal weight after years of struggling? Just stick with it, and as you start looking and feeling great, your friends and family may come around and want to do it with you.

I had a 58-year-old patient named Betty who had chronic migraines, vertigo, high blood pressure, digestive problems, and was overweight for many years. She was ready to give up at two weeks on the FreeDiet® because of all the pressure she was getting from her friends and family. Even her therapist told her she was crazy for doing it. Fortunately, she came in to see me, and I was able to give her some guidance and encouragement, so she stuck with it.

She continued to improve, losing 50 pounds in six months and normalizing her blood pressure. No more migraines, vertigo, chronic pain. She was able to avoid the recommended neck surgery, and her chronic digestive issues cleared up. By the way, she did all this while working in a bakery and still avoiding gluten, grains, sugar, yeast, eggs, and dairy.

Doesn't it cost a lot of money to eat like this?

Actually, eating like this can save you money. Even with buying high-quality organic produce, grass-fed meat, organic chicken, and wild fish. Preparing your meals at home, not eating out for lunch, not eating dinner in restaurants so often, not picking up your daily Starbucks, and not buying those packaged convenience foods can save you a lot of money.

How am I going to eat out at restaurants while on the FreeDiet®?

Select items such as beef, chicken, or seafood with vegetables. If it comes with potatoes, rice, or pasta, ask to substitute with an extra vegetable. Add a salad for an appetizer with olive oil and lemon. It is important to ask the server if the menu items you're interested in are gluten free, as many of the sauces, gravies, and marinades have gluten and other "avoid" items in them, like sugar, dairy, and vinegar.

How am I going to follow the FreeDiet® while traveling?

For breakfast, bring a shaker cup and pack all the powdered shake ingredients in individual Ziploc bags (or travel packs), one for each morning. Each morning, fill the shaker cup with water and all the ingredients, shake well, and there you go. That's your breakfast. If you can get a hotel room with a kitchenette area, that's even better, but not a necessity.

One of my patients, Ellen, is 56 years old and travels regularly for a living. She's done amazingly well on the FreeDiet®. She lost 20 pounds in three months, her lifelong migraines and vertigo resolved, her digestive issues (pain, bloating, gas, and constipation) resolved, her fatigue and insomnia are better, and her chronic pain is better. She managed all of this while traveling. Also, in three months, her autoimmune antibodies went from a very high level to normal!

When traveling, Ellen orders from Amazon/Whole Foods and has food delivered to her hotel room with a kitchenette. Her food delivery would be waiting for her when she arrived.

When she goes out for dinner, she asks the server to make sure her steak, chicken, or fish is plain and gluten free, and comes with plenty of vegetables and a salad. She has been able to make amazing progress doing the FreeDiet®, even while traveling extensively.

What about communion in church?

If it's an important part of your religious practice, then there are gluten-free hosts that are available. However, if communion is a casual thing for you, then it's best to be avoided during the FreeDiet® Phase 1 and Phase 2. The same goes for the wine or grape juice.

I saw a 38-year-old woman with chronic UTIs. She had been on antibiotics multiple times, but they kept returning. Then they had to use a catheter to apply the antibiotics and steroids directly in her bladder on many occasions, still with no success. After her initial evaluation and testing, two of the things she had were gluten sensitivity and yeast overgrowth/sensitivity. Once starting the FreeDiet®, her UTIs quickly cleared up until three months in when she had a major flare-up. This was right after consuming the bread and grape juice that she had at church one Sunday.

How can I possibly do the FreeDiet® if I'm vegan?

What you can do is use the organic pea protein for your FreeDiet® 3-Minute Super Smoothie. Instead of animal protein for lunch and dinner, use soaked nuts (see Chapter 3 or recipe chapter for instructions) like walnuts, pecans, macadamia nuts, cashews, hemp or pumpkin seeds instead.

One thing to keep in mind is that almost every vegan/vegetarian I have run lab tests on has been deficient in many nutrients, including vitamin B12, iron, and zinc.

No more excuses!

There are some characteristics that are important to being successful:

1. Do you really want to get better? Is there something or someone holding you back? Is there some benefit to you staying sick or overweight?
2. Do you believe you can get better? Has your disease become your identity? Do you spend hours a week on the internet identifying with your condition, reading about all the suffering people and the endless, confusing recommendations?
3. Do you feel you deserve to get better, or does everyone else come first in your life? Are you always putting yourself on the back burner and not taking the time for self-care?
4. Are you willing to commit, to invest in yourself and do what it takes to stay with it until you get better?

I found that if you have enough reasons why, you can overcome any challenge or excuse that comes up.

I had a 33-year-old patient named Autumn who was on 12 different medications. She had fatigue, pain, dizziness, insomnia, brain fog, skin issues, digestive issues, chronic bladder inflammation, interstitial cystitis, allergies, asthma, and even more. She felt so sick and miserable she was not able to work or even drive.

She improved so much in the first month on FreeDiet® that she was able to get off **all 12** prescription medications and function like an active person again. She said she was miserable for so long and started feeling so great doing the FreeDiet® that no food was worth going back to how miserable she felt before.

You can do this. You can stay the course, and you can get better! You can feel the best you have in years!

CHAPTER 5

THE FREEDIET® PHASE 2

Typically, you will stay on the FreeDiet® Phase 1 for 28 days. By this time, a lot of your symptoms should have improved considerably. You should have more energy, less pain, clearer thinking, improved focus and concentration, reduced excess fat, improved gut and skin issues, and be sleeping better.

Many of my patients tell me that they are feeling so good and losing weight for the first time in years, that they want to stay on FreeDiet® Phase 1 even longer. That's perfectly fine. For instance, one of my patients, a 56-year-old woman, stayed in Phase 1 for six months because her lifelong migraines and vertigo cleared up and she was sleeping through the night for the first time in years. She lost 25 pounds and was keeping it off very easily in FreeDiet® Phase 1.

After 28 days on Phase 1, you can look at your original health goals in Chapter 3 and write your percent improvement. Then retake the Health Assessment Quiz and total your score. You should be at least 50 percent better from where you started and well on your way to achieving all your health goals.

If you haven't seen a significant improvement, that usually means one of two things.

You did not follow it 100 percent, and you ate some "avoid" foods. This may even be accidental, like eating out and assuming what you're ordering is free of gluten.

If you HAVE followed it 100 percent, you may have other issues going on, like nutritional deficiencies, toxins, or infections.

In this case, you should get a proper evaluation and lab testing done to fig-ure out what else is going on. See Chapter 10 for more information on this.

One of my patients, a 30-year-old woman with acne, digestive symptoms, and fatigue, was doing much better after FreeDiet® Phase 1. However, she still had nagging rashes that weren't going away. After ordering a stool test, it came back positive for a parasite called blastocystis hominis. I treat-ed her with a three-month protocol (see Chapter 13 for details), retested her, and the parasite was gone, along with her skin issues.

Phase 2

Once you've completed the FreeDiet® Phase 1 and you are feeling better, you can go to the next phase. During FreeDiet® Phase 2, you can reintro-duce up to one new food every three days. Weigh yourself each morning upon arising. If you experience any symptoms or have gained over two pounds since the day before, avoid that food for another month before trying again.

Common food sensitivity reactions include:
- runny nose, sinus congestion, sneezing, postnasal drip, ear infections and/or clogging
- ear itching, eye redness and itching, crusty/sticky eyelids, canker sores
- chest congestion, coughing, asthma, shortness of breath
- abdominal pain, indigestion, reflux, bloating, gas, belching, diarrhea, constipation
- fatigue, sleepiness
- brain fog, lack of focus or concentration, hyperactivity
- depression, anxiety, moodiness
- headaches, migraines, dizziness
- heart palpitations, increased blood pressure
- skin reactions such as acne, canker sores, itching, eczema, rashes, dark circles under eyes

- genital itch or discharge
- numbness, tingling, stinging, burning
- joint or back pain, inflammation, swelling
- weight gain

A food reaction could also include a flare-up of any of the symptoms you had before you started the FreeDiet®.

If you started with one new food on Monday and you had no reaction that day, Tuesday, or Wednesday, then you can add this food back to your "allowed" eating list. You can then try another new food on Thursday, and so on. If you do react to a certain food, wait till those symptoms clear up before trying another food.

Start with **one food at a time**. I had a patient that was feeling great and lost 20 pounds during Phase 1. His chronic digestive problems and many other symptoms cleared up during this time. He was feeling so good that he decided he would go to a charity pancake breakfast. No big deal. It was only one time, right? While there, he ate eggs, sausage, and pancakes with syrup. When you include the coffee and orange juice he drank, that's at least six new foods at once!

Soon after, he had severe abdominal pain, vomiting, and diarrhea. Which of the foods caused it? He had no way of knowing (Not to mention, most of these foods aren't even in Phase 2.). **One food at a time!** You worked so hard to get this far, so stick with the program. This way, you can find out which foods may be bothersome for you.

I had another patient, a 36-year-old woman, who was feeling great after six weeks of FreeDiet® Phase 1. She lost 16 pounds, and her thyroid goiter had shrunk considerably. As she started adding foods back into her diet, she didn't feel well. It turns out that she was using a spice mix that included three of the spices in Phase 2. Which one was causing problems? No idea. I advised her to use individual spices initially to make sure she was okay with each of them.

In addition to this, many commercial spices (especially spice mixes) contain gluten, so you should make sure to buy gluten-free spices. If it doesn't say so on the bottle, check the company's website to see if they are certified gluten free.

The idea is to reintroduce food from the list below one at a time. Keep in mind that we are not adding back some foods until FreeDiet® Phase 3.

Foods to Reintroduce in Phase 2

In FreeDiet® Phase 2, you can reintroduce the foods in the chart below listed in bold. These are the new foods that you can add back, one at a time, every three days if you'd like. If there is any food that you know you are sensitive or allergic to, avoid it even if it's on the allowed list. Phase 1 foods are listed as well in regular text.

The FreeDiet® Phase 2

You may reintroduce up to one new food (in bold) every three days.

Food Groups	Allowed	Avoid
Proteins	Chicken and turkey (except ground), lamb, beef, bison, fish (salmon, sole, sardines, flounder, pollock, Atlantic cod, Atlantic mackerel), **eggs, pastured pork and bacon, wild scallops and shrimp, and other shellfish** Best choices: organic poultry, grass-fed beef and lamb, wild-caught fish	Barbecued or blackened meats, cold cuts, ham, hot dogs, sausage, ground chicken, ground turkey, smoked or canned meats and fish, bluefish, grouper, halibut, king mackerel, mahi-mahi, marlin, orange roughy, shark, swordfish, tilefish, tuna, sea bass, tilapia, imitation crab
Legumes	**Green beans, peas,** pea protein	All other beans, lentils, soybeans, tofu, miso, tempeh, alfalfa
Dairy	Organic: Ghee (clarified butter) **butter, cream, goat and sheep milk and cheese**	Cow milk and cheese, yogurt, kefir, cottage cheese, ice cream, non-dairy creamers

Starch/Grains	Squash (i.e. butternut, acorn, spaghetti squash) cauliflower rice, **sweet and Hannah potato, yams, arrowroot, tapioca, yuca (cassava)**	Gluten: wheat, rye, barley, malt, couscous, spelt, Kamut, oats, corn, rice, amaranth, tapioca, buckwheat, millet, quinoa, sorghum, teff, pasta, bread, toast, cookies, cake, chips, crackers, popcorn, white potato
Vegetables	Fresh or frozen (preferably organic): romaine lettuce, cucumbers, avocado, arugula, butter lettuce, radishes, fennel, celery, asparagus, artichoke, watercress, jicama Cooked: kale, collards, cabbage, broccoli, cauliflower, bok choy, Brussels sprouts, turnips, turnip greens, garlic, onion, chayote squash, rutabaga, organic yellow squash, and zucchini, **green beans, rhubarb, beet greens, callaloo, Swiss chard, spinach, eggplant, beets, carrots, parsnips, peppers, sunchoke (Jerusalem artichoke), tomatoes**	Corn, mushrooms, white potatoes, all canned or creamed vegetables Raw: kale, collards, cabbage, broccoli, cauliflower, bok choy, Brussels sprouts
Soups	Homemade soups with no bullion, **cream soups**	Canned or boxed soups
Fruits	Fresh and frozen fruit with no added sugar (preferably organic): blueberries, cherries, cranberries, lemon, lime, apricot, coconut, kiwi, peach, pear, plum, organic papaya, starfruit, pomegranate, apple, **orange, grapefruit, tangerine, mandarin orange, blackberries, raspberries, strawberries, ackee, banana, breadfruit, fresh figs, jackfruit, goji berry, soursop, mango, pineapple, plantain, grapes, cantaloupe, honeydew, watermelon** *1 serving/cup per day	Dried fruit such as raisins, figs, and dates; canned fruits
Fats/Oils,Nuts, and Seeds	Cold/expeller-pressed, unrefined, extra virgin olive and coconut oil; avocado oil; ground flaxseeds, hemp seeds Raw, soaked: walnuts, cashews, pecans, hazelnuts, macadamia nuts, Brazil nuts, pine nuts, chestnuts, pumpkin seeds, tiger nuts, **almonds, chia, sunflower and sesame seeds**	Margarine, shortening, refined oils, soy, corn and canola oil, mayonnaise, salad dressings, peanuts, pistachios, nut butter

Beverages	Filtered water, green tea (organic), homemade nut and coconut milk, **herbal tea** (gluten-free), **coffee** (organic), **cacao, coconut water** (max. 8 oz. which can replace one fruit)	Milk: cow, goat, soy, rice, almond; fruit juice and drinks, black tea, kombucha, alcohol, beer, wine, Champagne, soda, sports drinks, coconut water, seltzer, kefir, kombucha
Sweeteners	Stevia, monk fruit (lo han guo), **erythritol, xylitol (non-GMO birch)**	High fructose corn syrup, corn syrup, agave, rice syrup, white or brown sugar, cane sugar, dehydrated cane juice, malt, fruit juice concentrate, honey, molasses, dextrose, glucose, maple syrup, coconut sugar and nectar, aspartame, acesulfame K, saccharin, sucralose
Spices and condiments	Himalayan or sea salt, gluten-free herbs and spices including basil, oregano, thyme, cilantro, coriander, cumin, garlic, ginger, turmeric, lemongrass, mint, parsley, rosemary, sage, cinnamon, clove, vanilla **Black or white pepper, cayenne, chili powder, crushed red pepper, curry, nutmeg, paprika, coconut aminos, carob, gluten/sugar-free dark chocolate/cacao (like Lily's or Lakanto)**	Vinegar (all types), ketchup, mustard, relish, salsa, barbecue and steak sauce, soy and teriyaki sauce, miso, tempeh, tofu, canned foods, milk chocolate, olives, pickled and fermented foods, yeast containing products, nutritional and brewer's yeast (*saccharomyces cerevisiae*)

The FreeDiet® Food Reintroduction Chart

Here is a chart to keep track of the new foods you add back in the FreeDiet® Phase 2. If you would like to reintroduce new foods, add one new food every three days.

If you experience any symptoms, write the symptom and the severity in those columns. This way, you will end up with a list of certain foods, if any, that you have a reaction to.

If you experience any symptoms or gain over two pounds since the day before, avoid that food for at least another month before trying again. If you react to a certain food, wait until those symptoms clear up before trying another new food.

Day/Date	New Food	List symptoms, if any. These may include: runny nose, sinus congestion, sneezing, postnasal drip, ear infections and/or clogging ear itching, eye redness and itching, crusty/sticky eyelids, canker sores chest congestion, coughing, asthma, shortness of breath abdominal pain, indigestion, reflux, bloating, gas, belching, diarrhea, constipation fatigue, sleepiness brain fog, lack of focus or concentration, hyperactivity depression, anxiety, moodiness headaches, migraines, dizziness, vertigo heart palpitations, increased blood pressure skin reactions such as acne, canker sores, itching, eczema, rashes, dark circles under eyes genital itch or discharge numbness, tingling, stinging, burning joint or back pain, inflammation, swelling, weight gain	Score: 0 = none 1 = mild 2 = moderate 3 = severe	Morning Weight (lbs. or kg)
1				
2				
3				

4				
5				
6				
7				
8				
9				
10				
11				
12				
13				
14				
15				
16				
17				
18				
19				
20				
21				
22				
23				
24				
25				
26				
27				
28				
29				
30				
31				
32				
33				
34				
35				
36				
37				
38				
39				
40				
41				
42				

The FreeDiet® Phase 2 Shopping List

Proteins
- Beef, grass-fed
- Bison, grass-fed
- Lamb, grass-fed
- Chicken, preferably organic (not ground)
- Turkey, preferably organic (not ground)
- Fish: wild salmon, sole, flounder, sardines, pollock, Atlantic cod, Atlantic mackerel
- Eggs
- Pastured pork and bacon
- Wild scallops, shrimp, and other shellfish

Vegetables (preferably organic)
- Artichoke
- Arugula
- Avocado (fruit)
- Butter lettuce
- Celery
- Cucumbers
- Fennel
- Jicama
- Radishes
- Romaine lettuce
- Watercress
- Beets
- Carrots
- Parsnips
- Peppers
- Sunchokes
- Tomatoes

For cooking:
- Acorn squash
- Asparagus
- Bok choy
- Broccoli
- Brussels sprouts
- Butternut squash
- Cabbage
- Cauliflower
- Chayote squash
- Collards
- Garlic
- Kale
- Onion
- Rutabaga

- Spaghetti squash
- Starfruit
- Turnips
- Turnip greens
- Yellow squash, organic
- Zucchini, organic
- Green beans
- Peas

- Rhubarb
- Beet greens
- Callaloo
- Swiss chard
- Spinach
- Green beans
- Eggplant

Starches

- Sweet potato
- Hannah potato
- Yam

- Yuca (cassava)
- Tapioca
- Arrowroot

Fruits (preferably organic)

- Apple
- Apricot
- Blueberries
- Cherries
- Coconut
- Kiwi
- Lemon
- Lime
- Papaya, organic
- Peach
- Pear
- Plum
- Pomegranate
- Starfruit
- Ackee
- Banana
- Blackberries
- Breadfruit

- Cantaloupe
- Fresh figs
- Goji berry
- Grapefruit
- Grapes
- Honeydew
- Jackfruit
- Mandarin orange
- Mango
- Orange
- Pineapple
- Plantain
- Raspberries
- Soursop
- Strawberries
- Tangerine
- Watermelon

Dairy (organic)
- Ghee (clarified butter)
- Butter
- Cream
- Goat and sheep cheese
- Goat and sheep milk

Oils (cold/expeller-pressed, unrefined, extra virgin, preferably organic)
- Avocado oil
- Coconut oil
- Ghee (clarified butter)
- Olive oil

Nuts/Seeds (preferably raw and organic)
- Brazil nuts
- Cashews
- Chestnuts
- Flaxseeds
  (for grinding at home) or
- Ground flaxseeds
- Hazelnuts
- Hemp seeds
- Macadamia nuts
- Pecans
- Pine nuts
- Pumpkin seeds
- Tiger nuts
- Walnuts
- Almonds
- Chia seeds
- Sesame seeds
- Sunflower seeds

Beverages
- Filtered water
- Green tea, organic
- Herbal tea (gluten-free)
- Cacao
- Coconut water
- Coffee, organic

Sweeteners
- Stevia
- Monk fruit (lo han guo)
- Erythritol
- Xylitol (non-GMO birch)

Spices (preferably organic)
- Basil
- Chives
- Cilantro
- Cinnamon
- Cloves
- Coriander
- Cumin
- Dill weed

- Garlic
- Ginger
- Himalayan or sea salt
- Lemongrass
- Mace
- Mint
- Onion powder
- Oregano
- Parsley
- Peppermint
- Rosemary
- Saffron
- Sage
- Spearmint
- Thyme
- Turmeric
- Vanilla (not vanillin)
- Black or white pepper
- Cayenne
- Chili powder
- Crushed red pepper
- Curry
- Nutmeg
- Paprika
- Coconut aminos
- Carob
- Dark chocolate/cacao (gluten/sugar-free, i.e. Lily's or Lakanto)

Frozen Foods (preferably organic)

- Blueberries
- Cherries
- Artichokes
- Asparagus
- Broccoli
- Brussels sprouts
- Cauliflower
- Cauliflower rice
- Collards
- Kale
- Blackberries
- Raspberries
- Strawberries
- Green beans
- Peas
- Spinach

CHAPTER 6

THE FREEDIET® PHASE 3

By now, you should be continuing to feel better and have had success with weight loss, if that was your goal. Update your Health Goals and Health Assessment Quiz from Chapter 3. Compare your current score to the Initial and Phase 1 results. You should have continued to improve in both areas.

After going through FreeDiet® Phase 2, you should have a list of foods you are fine with and a list of foods that may have caused some issues. FreeDiet® Phase 3 is the "maintenance" phase. You will soon have a customized diet based on your unique body chemistry, specific for you, as opposed to a one-size-fits-all diet.

A 44-year-old patient named Gina had chronic sinus problems her whole life. She had to take daily medications just to make it through the day. Her sinuses cleared up while on the FreeDiet® Phase 1, and she was finally able to ditch her sinus medications. In the FreeDiet® Phase 2, she found out that every time she ate eggs, her sinuses would flare up—not dairy, but eggs.

Each person has different reactive foods. As the Roman philosopher, Lucretius expressed in 55 B.C., "That which to some is food, to others is rank poison."

In FreeDiet® Phase 3, you can add additional foods from the Phase 3 list, one at a time every few days and record your reactions. Only do this if you're feeling good and most of your symptoms have cleared up. Only then are you ready to try out foods that may be more reactive.

In the FreeDiet® Phase 3 chart, you will see the allowed foods in the left column. The new foods you can add are in bold. Again, up to one new food every three days. The next column is the "always avoid" column, as these foods are just not good for you at all.

You'll see under starch/grains in the avoid column that gluten is listed. I believe most people would do best to continue to avoid it. The exception might be if you are feeling good and you have no digestive issues, autoimmune conditions, skin or thyroid issues, pain, memory and concentration problems, etc. However, even then, gluten could still be doing hidden damage. Gluten is known to cause increased intestinal permeability (leaky gut), which can be a trigger for autoimmune conditions.

I've tested many patients for gluten sensitivity, and almost everyone tests positive. Many have positive Celiac genes. I don't even remember the last time that I recommended someone go back to eating gluten. The same goes for grains in general, as they tend to be inflammatory. Yes, even the non-gluten grains like oats, corn, rice, and quinoa.

Yeast is another issue for a lot of people, so I continue to recommend avoiding kombucha, alcohol, beer, wine, soda, fruit drinks, and sports drinks. If yeast is not an issue for you (and, of course, you are of legal drinking age) you can first reintroduce limited amounts of non-gluten alcohol like vodka, tequila, or rum and see how you do. In general, though, I'm not a big fan of any of the above products.

Sugar is another substance that should continue to be avoided because of its inflammatory nature. It also feeds yeast and other microbes. This is why I recommend you continue to avoid fruit drinks, dried fruits, and other types of sugar. I recommend limiting fruit servings to two servings per day and getting your phytonutrients from eating plenty of vegetables.

The other thing with sugar, gluten, and yeast is that if you start eating them a little you can get your cravings back. Before you know it, you want it all the time, making it difficult to stop, and your symptoms can creep back.

I had a 61-year-old patient named Tom who, with the FreeDiet®, was able to resolve his fatigue, neuropathy, dizziness, shortness of breath, back and joint pain. Within four weeks, he decreased his blood pressure 35 points and cholesterol 65 points both down to normal and raised his testosterone 227 points (51 percent) to optimal levels. He did this without medication and lost 11 pounds in that first month.

Amongst other things, he was highly gluten sensitive and had yeast overgrowth, but over the holidays started eating gluten foods and drinking wine. Of course, he didn't stop on just one occasion. On his next evaluation, his testosterone decreased 42 percent, and his high blood pressure returned.

Then he got back on the FreeDiet® and at his follow-up visit two months later, he was fine again. What was remarkable was that he was able to increase his testosterone by 95 percent (371 points) in those two months without taking hormones.

This demonstrates how important it is to avoid those inflammatory foods that are wreaking havoc on your system. So be careful about adding foods back you know you are sensitive to.

If you haven't improved considerably through the FreeDiet® Phase 1 and Phase 2, I would have your doctor look into other root causes like deficiencies, toxins, infections, and hormones. See Chapter 10 for more details.

Allergy and Sensitivity Testing

I've found that most people going through the phases of the FreeDiet® do fine with discovering what foods they do well with, and which are problematic. If you still have symptoms and want to get even more specific, food allergy and/or sensitivity testing can be a good option. You can see Chapter 10 for more information as well.

The downside of food sensitivity testing is that the test itself can be useless without proper interpretation. For example, I had a very obese patient who previously ordered a test through her doctor and didn't have any guidance except for the test results along with the recommended diet that came with it. She did not lose one pound, nor did any of her many symptoms improve following it. That's because she was eating loads of the allowed grains and high-sugar foods and wasn't looking at the whole picture.

It's best used with the FreeDiet® as the foundation and then to see what other foods you may be reactive to that are allowed—such as flaxseeds or lemon—not which foods you are okay with, because there can be a lot of false negatives. Especially if you haven't eaten the food in a while.

Another downside is that some food tests are not accurate or reliable. I've used several labs over the past 33-plus years on myself and many patients and have found certain labs much more accurate than others. The ones I recommend test for food sensitivities with more than one type of antibody reaction. As opposed to measuring only the IgG antibodies, I prefer tests that simultaneously measure various types of delayed sensitivity reactions.

Then there are tests for food allergies, which cause reactions immediately, or certainly within two hours. An example would be peanuts causing hives, difficulty breathing, swelling, itchy throat, abdominal pain, and/or vomiting. If a true food allergy is suspected, then an IgE food allergy blood panel would be recommended.

Food sensitivities are harder to figure out than allergies because they are delayed reactions. It could be a few hours up to three days until you notice any symptoms. That's why I have you add one new food every three days. These symptoms may include a runny nose, sinus congestion, sneezing, postnasal drip, brain fog, headaches, heart palpitations, abdominal pain, indigestion, bloating, gas, belching, diarrhea, constipation, fatigue, numbness, tingling, burning, joint or back pain, and skin reactions such as acne, canker sores, itching, eczema, a rash, and other symptoms.

A 74-year-old patient named Meryl came to me with digestive symptoms and chronic knee pain. Her doctors said that due to her severe arthritis, she needed a knee replacement. She didn't want to do that. Besides doing physical treatment, I did some testing and found out she had a gluten sensitivity. Between going on the FreeDiet® and the Natural Medicine Formulas, along with chiropractic care, soft tissue treatment, laser, and functional exercises, she got to a point where she had no pain whatsoever. Even with severe arthritis that she had in her knee joint.

After weeks with no pain, Meryl came in for an appointment and said she woke up with severe knee pain that made it difficult to walk. The conversation went like this:

Me: Well, did you do anything differently yesterday?
Meryl: No, not at all.
Me: Did you eat anything different?
Meryl: No.
Me: Anything with gluten in it?
Meryl: No.
Me: Well, what did you have for dinner last night?
Meryl: Oh, I had an avocado sandwich with Ezekiel bread.
Me: Well, don't you know that Ezekiel bread has gluten in it?
Meryl: It does?

After a couple of days of avoiding of gluten and grains, her pain went away again. Meryl's story is an example of food sensitivity as opposed to an allergy. That's why it's so important to figure out what foods you're sensitive to that are causing your underlying health issues.

So, as you are adding foods throughout FreeDiet® Phase 3, make sure you write them down in the Food Reintroduction Chart you started in Phase 2. By the end, you should end up with an expanded list of foods that your body is okay with and a list of foods you're not okay with. You will have a diet that is specific for you, as opposed to a one-size-fits-all diet.

The FreeDiet® Phase 3

You may reintroduce up to 1 new food every 3 days

Food Groups	Allowed	Avoid	Use minimally if at all
Proteins	Chicken and turkey (except ground), lamb, beef, bison, fish (salmon, sole, sardines, flounder, pollock, Atlantic cod, Atlantic mackerel), eggs, pastured pork and bacon, wild scallops and shrimp and other shellfish Best choices: organic poultry, grass-fed beef and lamb, wild-caught fish	Blackened meats, conventional cold cuts, pork, hot dogs and sausage, imitation crab	Smoked, barbe-cued or canned meats and fish, bluefish, grouper, halibut, king mack-erel, mahi-mahi, marlin, orange roughy, shark, swordfish, tilefish, tuna, sea bass, tilapia, ground chicken and turkey, gluten-free sausage and hot dogs
Legumes	Green beans, peas, pea protein, **garbanzo beans (chickpeas), hummus, alfalfa sprouts**	soybeans, tofu, miso, tempeh, soy milk	All other beans, lentils
Dairy	Organic: Ghee (clarified butter) butter, cream, goat and sheep milk and cheese	Traditional non-dairy creamers	Cow milk and cheese, yogurt, kefir (no added sugar), cottage cheese, ice cream
Starch/ Grains	Squash (i.e. butternut, acorn, spaghetti squash) cauliflower rice, sweet and Hannah potato, yams, chickpea pasta, arrow-root, tapioca, yuca (cassava), **white potato**	Gluten: wheat, rye, barley, malt, couscous, spelt, Kamut, oats, rice, millet, pasta, bread, toast, cookies, cake, chips, crackers, corn and popcorn	amaranth, buck-wheat, quinoa, sorghum, teff, organic corn and popcorn, wild rice

Vegetables	Fresh or frozen (preferably organic): romaine lettuce, cucumbers, avocado, arugula, butter lettuce, radishes, fennel, celery, asparagus, watercress, jicama Cooked: kale, collards, cabbage, broccoli, cauliflower, bok choy, Brussels sprouts, turnips, turnip greens, garlic, onion, chayote squash, rutabaga, organic yellow squash and zucchini, green beans, rhubarb, beet greens, callaloo, Swiss chard, spinach, eggplant, beets, carrots, parsnips, peppers, sunchoke (Jerusalem artichoke), tomatoes, **mushrooms**	Corn, canned or creamed vegetables	<p>Organic corn</p> Raw: kale, spinach, collards, cabbage, broccoli, cauliflower, bok choy, Brussels sprouts
Soups	Homemade soups with no bullion, cream soups	Canned or boxed soups	
Fruits	Fresh and frozen fruit with no added sugar (preferably organic): blueberries, cherries, apple, lemons, limes, peaches, pears, plums, coconut, pomegranate, starfruit, orange, grapefruit, tangerine, mandarin orange, blackberries, raspberries, strawberries, ackee, banana, breadfruit, fresh figs, jackfruit, goji berry, soursop, mango, pineapple, plantain, grapes, cantaloupe, honeydew, watermelon ***1–2 servings/day**	Canned fruits	Dried fruit such as raisins, figs, and dates
Fats/Oils, Nuts, and Seeds	Cold/expeller-pressed, unrefined, extra virgin olive and coconut oil, avocado oil; ground flaxseeds, hemp seeds, Raw, soaked: walnuts, cashews, pecans, hazelnuts, macadamia nuts, Brazil nuts, pine nuts, chestnuts, pumpkin seeds, tiger nuts, almonds, chia, sunflower and sesame seeds, **nut butter, avocado oil mayonnaise**	Margarine, shortening, refined oils, soy, corn and canola oil, mayonnaise, commercial salad dressings	Pistachios, peanuts

Beverages	Filtered water, green tea (organic), homemade nut and coconut milk, herbal tea (gluten-free), coffee (organic), cacao, coconut water (max 8 oz. can replace 1 fruit), **black tea, nut/coconut milk with no added sugar**	Soy and rice milk, fruit drinks, alcohol, beer, soda, sports drinks	Cow's milk, fruit juice, seltzer, kefir (no added sugar), kombucha, wine, Champagne, gluten-free alcohol (certain vodkas, rum, tequila, etc.)
Sweeteners	Stevia, monk fruit (lo han guo), erythritol, xylitol (non-GMO birch), **very small amounts: honey, molasses, non-GMO dextrose, glucose, real maple syrup, coconut sugar and nectar**	High fructose corn syrup, corn syrup, agave, rice syrup, white or brown sugar, malt, pancake syrup, fruit juice concentrate, aspartame, acesulfame K, saccharin, sucralose	Cane sugar, dehydrated cane juice
Spices and condiments	Himalayan or sea salt, gluten-free herbs and spices including basil, oregano, thyme, cilantro, coriander, cumin, garlic, ginger, turmeric, lemongrass, mint, parsley, rosemary, sage, cinnamon, clove, vanilla Black or white pepper, cayenne, chili pepper, curry, nutmeg, paprika, red pepper, coconut aminos, carob, gluten/sugar-free dark chocolate/cacao (like Lily's or Lakanto), **olives, pickled and fermented foods, apple cider vinegar**	soy and teriyaki sauce, miso, tempeh, tofu	Yeast containing products, nutritional and brewer's yeast (*saccharomyces cerevisiae*), canned foods, vinegar, ketchup, mustard, mayonnaise, relish, barbecue and steak sauce, milk chocolate

CHAPTER 7

THE FREEDIET® SUPPLEMENTS: NATURAL MEDICINE FORMULAS®

Do you need to take vitamin supplements?

After I graduated from Rutgers University, I moved into an apartment. My new roommate was taking lots of different vitamin supplements. I thought he was crazy with all those bottles. After all, I studied physiology and nutrition extensively in school and was taught that you could get all your nutrients from food. They taught us that supplements just create expensive urine, or at most—and this is the exception—you may need to take a "one-a-day" multivitamin from the drugstore. You know, those rock-hard colored tablets.

Meanwhile, my roommate was quite healthy, very muscular, and in shape, while I was tired and in pain all the time. What I realized on my journey since then was that I, in fact, was deficient in many nutrients, including magnesium, vitamin B12, vitamin D, and others. My roommate was right all along, and despite my better education, I was the one who was mistaken.

You've probably heard that a balanced diet is all you need to get all your nutrients. However, I find that is not the case at all. There are certain factors like stress, medications, exercise, and sweating that increase your need for vitamins, minerals, and antioxidants. After testing thousands of patients over the past 33-plus years. I have to say it's rare that I find a patient that is not deficient in various nutrients. Also, digestive issues can cause malabsorption that further increases your need for vitamins and minerals.

Overall, the answer to that question is yes. I do believe you need to take nutritional supplements.

Which ones do you need to take?

There is what I call the Functional Five because they are the basic nutrients that most everyone needs for keeping your body functioning at the highest level. These include a multivitamin, fish oil, magnesium, vitamin D, and probiotics.

Functional Five supplements:

ActivMulti™ w/o iron—multivitamin

OmegaSorb3X™—fish oil capsules

D3 5000 + K2—most need 5000 IU/day of vitamin D

Magnesium Malate (or Citrate if you have constipation)

ProbioSupreme™ 30—probiotic

It's important to take only high-quality supplements. There are a wide variety of supplements available out there—some are excellent, some are okay, and some are terrible. After trying hundreds of different supplements over the last 33-plus years, I've come up with a line of supplements that I know are effective based on clinical experience and thousands of pre- and post-lab testing of patients.

Of course, you don't have to use my supplements but I do recommend our Natural Medicine Formulas line for many reasons. It is a pharmaceutical-grade professional line of supplements that is very high-quality and offers excellent absorption. They are free of chemical preservatives, artificial colorings, gluten, and other common allergens. The manufacturers I use meet or exceed GMP (Good Manufacturing Practices) standards.

We use bioavailable nutrients like methyl folate instead of folic acid, as many people have what they call an MTHFR gene mutation, which prevents them from breaking down folic acid. Taking folic acid can be more harmful for these people than not taking anything. Taking methyl folate, however, bypasses that step and allows you to utilize it in your body.

We looked at the balance of the various nutrients, like the balance between calcium and magnesium. We also considered the risks of taking a multivitamin with iron if you don't need iron—which can then be toxic to your system. Also, having chelated minerals versus inorganic minerals is very important for absorption reasons.

Absorption is so important with vitamin supplements. A patient once told me her father-in-law had his septic tank cleaned out, and afterward the technician asked him how long he had been taking vitamins.

He said he took a multivitamin daily for many years—one of those rock-hard, heavily advertised, brightly-colored multi's you get at the supermarket or pharmacy.

"Why do you ask?"

"There were thousands of tablets at the bottom of your septic tank!"

And he thought he was saving money by buying cheap vitamins.

As you can see, there are many things to consider when choosing supplements. Dosing is very important as well. For instance, I had a patient who was taking vitamin D that she bought off the internet. She was taking one *dropper* instead of one *drop*. Turns out she was taking 50,000 units a day for many months—and she was pregnant! She was vomiting every single day through her eighth month of pregnancy. When she first came in, I ran her lab tests and discovered she had vitamin D toxicity. I had her stop taking it, and the vomiting resolved immediately. By the next day, she was able to stop taking her prescription medication for morning sickness.

Beyond the Functional Five, there are specific needs that you may have. After testing thousands of patients, the most common extra supplements that I see patients needing are vitamin B12, iron, and zinc, in addition to magnesium and vitamin D.

Vitamin B12 deficiency can cause neurological issues, such as brain fog, loss of memory and concentration, numbness, tingling, and fatigue.

Low iron can cause fatigue, weakness, shortness of breath, restless leg syndrome, lack of focus and concentration, dizziness, heart palpitations, cold hands and feet, brittle nails, and hair loss.

Most every patient I see has digestive issues, so invariably I initially recommend digestive enzymes. The most common one I recommend is GastricZyme™, which contains stomach enzymes that many people are low in. It contains betaine HCl and pepsin, along with gentian root, which promote healthy digestion, especially of proteins. It supports the absorption of micronutrients and helps stimulate the flow of bile and pancreatic enzymes, which break down carbohydrates, fats, and protein.

I recommend taking most supplements with meals as opposed to after. If you're taking five to ten different supplements, take them one or two at a time at the beginning or throughout the meal instead of taking all of them after your meal. Probiotics, magnesium, and certain other supplements can be taken between meals as an option.

Aren't good supplements very expensive?

It may seem like that. However, with the quality, bioavailability, and therapeutic dosing, it can actually be very good value. A patient asked me recently if she could take a fish oil supplement that was bought online. It was very cheap and from a popular, well-respected company. When I looked at it, I discovered that although it was one-fourth the price of our fish oil supplements, it took nine capsules of theirs to equal the dose in only one of ours. What she thought was saving her money was actually costing her more to pay less.

Oftentimes the supplements from the supermarket, drugstore, big-box chains, and online have other ingredients in them that make them unacceptable in the FreeDiet®. They may include gluten, yeast, aluminum, dyes, and other things that you wouldn't want to put into your body.

There is a popular children's multivitamin that contains the artificial sweetener aspartame, sugar, corn syrup, aluminum, hydrogenated vegetable oils, and so on. Cheap, yes, but at what cost to your child's health?

How long do you need to take supplements?

For most people, I recommend taking the Functional Five indefinitely. And for other supplements, it depends on your condition and lab test results. Iron needs, for instance, are determined from lab testing. Depending on your levels, you may need to take a certain dosage and then do follow-up lab testing until your iron levels get to a certain point. Then you would reduce your intake or discontinue.

The same idea holds true with vitamin B12 deficiency or iodine. If someone has thyroid nodules or goiter and testing reveals an iodine deficiency, I would have them take a certain amount until testing reveals they need a lower dose or don't need it anymore.

Why would I need to take vitamin D if I go out in the sun?

I thought this, too. I live in south Florida, and years ago, I lived at the beach and was out in the sun two or three times a week. I checked my vitamin D level, and it was extremely low, which shocked me. It seemed that my olive complexion and easy tanning was decreasing my ability to utilize vitamin D from sunshine.

At the time, among many other health challenges, I had chronic upper back pain. No matter what treatment I received, the pain was there all the time. However, when I started taking 5,000 IU of vitamin D per day to increase my level up to normal, I noticed my back pain went away. I wasn't even thinking at the time that it would happen. I just noticed after doing it for a while and put two and two together. Yes, vitamin D deficiency can cause chronic pain.

Another time, I had a patient fly in from the islands to see me. He was a Bahamian gardener who worked out in the sun 40 hours per week and had fatigue and chronic pain. I checked, and he was also deficient in vitamin D! The fact is the darker your skin, the more difficult it is to produce vitamin D from the sun.

Overall, I recommend you take the Functional Five, and if you're able to, get tested for your vitamin and mineral levels and see what else you might need. Refer to Chapter 10 for the specific lab testing to do that.

Along with the proper diet, taking high-quality vitamin and mineral supplements can dramatically improve your health and help you feel the best you have in years!

CHAPTER 8

THE FREEDIET® FITNESS

How would you like to learn a simple 20-minute routine that can burn fat and tone your body?

This is not your typical old-school cardio where you spend hours in the gym and on the treadmill. This is fast, efficient, and effective.

Over the years, I have had many new patients come in that were very overweight, yet insisted they were exercising regularly without being able to lose a single pound.

Some of them were training for a road race, half marathon, or triathlon. We're talking hours a week of doing endurance training and not losing a pound. How is this possible? After all, they were burning all those extra calories.

The truth is that long bouts of slow cardio do not work. You may lose muscle tone, deplete your hormones, or stress your adrenals, and it doesn't burn fat very well at all. Not to mention the injuries from overuse, including heel spurs, plantar fasciitis, shin splints, knee pain, and low back pain, to name a few. Long, slow endurance exercise can also weaken your immune system, resulting in more colds and sickness.

What's even worse is that many people doing endurance training are drinking those awful sugary sports drinks, goops, and gels loaded with chemicals.

High-intensity interval training (HIIT) or fast cardio is the way to go. It involves a three-minute warmup followed by 30 second sprints and a 90-second walk, jog, or slow pace. You repeat that cycle eight times, then you do a three-minute cooldown. This HIIT is from Dr. Joe Mercola and has amazing results.

When I first started doing this some years ago, I noticed I had more energy and was feeling better mentally, physically, and emotionally within a few short weeks. Within six weeks, I noticed more definition in my legs and glutes. Overall, I became much more muscular.

In the past, I would do phases of cardio, such as distance running, Stair-Master, or elliptical. I even did rollerblading for years when that was popular. It was so boring to be on the elliptical for 30–60 minutes at the same pace, and frankly, I never noticed much of a difference with any of these.

As a result, for quite some time I didn't do any cardio and only did resistance training at the gym. Once I found out about HIIT, I started doing it three times per week with amazing results. I gained ten pounds of muscle, which I had been unable to do for years.

The benefits of HIIT are an improvement in cardiovascular function, fat metabolism, hormones, energy, and muscle tone. Think about the sprinters in the Olympics. They are very toned and muscular versus a distance or marathon runner.

HIIT can be done either sprinting outside, on a stationary bike, or the elliptical. I do not recommend the treadmill, as it is easy to get injured while sprinting. The stationary bike is not the best either, as you don't get the benefits of a whole-body workout.

Sprinting outside is great if you can run without getting injured and you don't have any joint issues. Personally, I like the elliptical the best as it is very easy on your joints. Unlike running, there is no pounding on your feet, ankles, knees, hips, and lower back. It's a very smooth and effective full-body workout. I prefer the Precor EFX Elliptical Fitness Crosstrainer (see Resources section in the back) without the moving arm handles. This way you can keep your arms freely moving at your side as if you're sprinting in place. Visit nmcwellness.com/get-fit-burn-fat-with-hiit-elliptical/ to see how easy this is.

Strength Training

Do you really want to spend hours in the gym lifting weights? If you are like me, the answer is no. I like fast, efficient, challenging workouts that last 20–30 minutes or less. I say this after spending years in the gym with regular one-hour-plus workouts.

Watch this video at nmcwellness.com/home-exercises-for-strength-balance-video for a functional fitness routine that you can do very easily at home. All you need is an exercise ball and some bands.

Here are some of the exercises:

Squats

Hold on to a doorway or other stationary object and then sit back until your thighs are parallel with the floor. Hold for two seconds and rise slowly to just short of full extension. This way you avoid locking your knees, as you keep them slightly bent at the top of the movement.

You should be able to work your way up to 20 repetitions. As it gets easier, you can even do single-leg squats where you raise your heel on one side so you're putting most of the weight on the foot that is doing the pressing. Or you can put your non-weight-bearing foot in front of you.

Calf raises

Stand on the floor or on the edge of a step with your heels hanging off. Press up and let down slowly for 10 reps, then do 10 reps each leg.

Standing rows with resistance tubing

Holding both handles, start with arms straight with resistance tubing taught and fixed at one end.

Keep palms facing each other at mid-waist level, and pull for 10 to 15 reps.

Then, palms down with arms at chest level, pull for 10 to 15 reps.

Triceps extension

With resistance tubing and elbows bent, palms facing up, extend arms down. Hold for one second, then slowly back up. 10 to 15 reps.

Chest press

Push forward both arms and/or a single arm, with resistance tubing. 10 to 15 reps.

Biceps curls

With resistance tubing, flex arms 10 to 15 reps. Stepping on the tubing with both feet instead of one increases the resistance. Make sure the tubing is under the middle of your feet to prevent the band from sliding out and snapping up.

Lift and Press

Lift weighted ball off the floor and press overhead. 10 to 15 reps.

Band Pull Apart

With resistance tubing, external rotation and shoulder retraction with both arms. 10 to 15 reps.

Standing with elbows bent at sides, hold tubing taut in front of you in each hand and pull apart, bringing your shoulders back.

Back

Superman on the ball, both arms at once: On knees with abdomen on ball, extend torso with arms out at sides. 10 reps.

Superman on the ball with alternating arms: Same as above with one arm raising up overhead while the opposite thigh and leg extends up, then alternate. 10 reps.

Abdominals

Crunches on the ball: back on ball, hands behind head, elbows back, raise chest up until you feel abdomen tighten (suck abdomen at the beginning of each rep and hold in). 10 to 20 reps.

Obliques on the ball: five reps each side, same as above with moving right elbow toward right knee and then switch sides.

Pelvic tilts on the ball: back on ball, raise pelvis up, hold one second. 10 to 15 reps.

Planks: elbows on ball, suck abdomen in and flatten back, head straight. Hold for 30 seconds.

Stretching

Hold each for five seconds and do five reps:

Knee to chest: lay on back, bring one knee to chest with both hands, then switch sides.

Glutes: lay on back, bend right knee and place foot on floor across left knee, then pull right knee across, stretching the right gluteal area. Do five reps, then switch.

Piriformis: same as glutes only pull knee and ankle toward opposite shoulder.

Cat and dog: on hands and knees, flex and extend spine. Hold one second for five reps.

Up dog/child's pose: on hands and knees, drop abdomen to floor, keeping arms straight and extending spine. Then sit back on knees, flexing spine and looking down.

Upper spinal twist: on side, knees up, together, arms out in front, reach top arm over and touch opposite side of floor with back of hand.

Hip flexor stretch on one knee: on a mat or cushion with other foot on floor in front, flex pelvis and slowly lunge forward.

Side stretch: standing, lean to one side, then the other.

Neck range of motion: forward, back (mildly), lean to right and left, then look to right and left.

Shoulder retractions: arms at side, bring shoulders back. Hold one second for five reps.

Pec stretch: hand against wall at eye level, arm straight, rotate torso away while extending the other arm back.

Calf stretch: standing, one foot forward of the other, and lunge forward with back leg straight.

Quadriceps stretch: standing on left leg, hold on for balance if needed, hold right ankle with right hand and pull back and up. Do five reps and switch sides.

Hamstring stretch: left leg straight in front, right leg back, while holding on to a chair with left hand for balance, bend forward and touch left lower leg or foot with right hand. Do five reps and switch sides.

Strength Exercises	Reps	Sets
Squats: double work up to single	10–15	1–2
Calf raises: double work up to single	10–15	1–2
Rows: Low, palms in	10–15	1–2
Rows: High, palms down	10–15	1–2
Triceps Extensions, palms up	10–15	1–2
Chest Press	10–15	1–2
Biceps Curls	10–15	1–2
Band Pull-Apart	10–15	1–2
Shoulder retractions w/bands	10–15	1–2
Shoulder: abduct to 45 degrees w/ bands	10–15	1–2
Lift and Press Up	10–15	1–2

Strength Exercises	Reps	Sets
Plank	1	Hold for 30–60 seconds
Balance on one leg with pads	1	Hold for 30–60 seconds
Ball Exercises		
Ball Hug	5	1
Back Extensions on Ball	10	1
Extensions w/alt. R/L arms and legs	10	1
Crunches, vacuum (suck abdomen in)	10–20	1
Obliques	5 each side	1
Pelvic Tilts	10–15	1
Neck Extensions	10	1
Ball Stretch, resting head on ball	1	Hold for 20 seconds

Stretching Exercises	Repetitions	Hold for
Knee to chest	5	5 seconds
Glutes	5	5 seconds
Piriformis	5	5 seconds
Cat and dog	5	1 second
Up dog/child's pose	5	5 seconds
Upper spinal twist	5	5 seconds
Hip flexor stretch on knee	5	5 seconds
Side stretch	5	1 second
Neck range of motion	5	1 second
Shoulder retractions	5	1 second
Pec stretch, hand against wall	5	5 seconds
Hamstring: single leg	5	5 seconds
Calf stretch	5	5 seconds
Quadriceps stretch	5	5 seconds

CHAPTER 9

THE FREEDIET® LIFESTYLE —FREE FOR LIFE

Besides diet and supplements, there are many lifestyle changes you can make so that you can look and feel your best.

Stress management is a big one. We all know how much of a negative impact stress can have on your life. Stress is not a negative thing; it's merely the body's response to change. This could be physical, chemical, or mental stress. You cannot eliminate stress; it's simply a part of our everyday life. Instead, we're going to talk about ways you can handle stress much better.

Exercise is a great stress reliever. Even just taking a walk 15–30 minutes a day works wonders. I know you're busy, so you'll have to carve out time in your daily schedule to do this. If you spend 20–30 minutes doing exercise, you're not losing that time. You will usually get more than that back in terms of increased productivity throughout the day.

Getting out in nature is also a great way to relieve stress and clear your mind. Whether it's going to the beach, mountains, park, hiking in the woods or by a lake, or gardening in your backyard, these can help tremendously to ease the tension and help you feel rejuvenated. Breathing fresh air is an added benefit.

Spending time in the sun is also helpful. Of course, you want to avoid getting sunburn, but getting moderate amounts of sun can have benefits in improving your vitamin D levels as well as being a great stress reliever and rejuvenator.

Breathing. Stress can cause you to have short, shallow breaths. This can increase tension in your diaphragm muscle, reduce your oxygen, and raise your CO_2 levels. One thing you can do for this is take ten slow, deep diaphragmatic breaths, twice per day. That means when you inhale, you expand your lower abdomen, and upon exhaling, you suck in your abdomen. Breathe in through your nose for four seconds and breathe out through your mouth for eight seconds, ten times, slowly. Doing it outside in the fresh air is even better.

Prayer and meditation are great stress relievers. Just like with exercise, you may have not had the time to do this daily. I was experiencing the same thing for many years. Although I knew it was helpful, I found it hard to create a habit of setting aside 20 minutes a day solely dedicated to this.

I signed up for a meditation course where I had to take three classes in a row and then some weekly follow-up classes over six weeks. It was a small group, so there was accountability every time you went, and you had to tell everyone how it was going. Of course, having invested the time and money and having some accountability really allowed me to establish a daily habit.

Since then, I automatically do it because the routine has been established, and it has made a world of difference. The daily 20 minutes I spend in meditation and prayer result in my gaining much more time throughout the day in focus, concentration, and productivity.

Sleep. Getting a good night's sleep is one of the most important lifestyle habits you can have. If you're not getting seven to eight hours of a good night's sleep, it can lead to sleep deprivation, which can contribute to:
- Fatigue
- Brain fog: lack of focus and concentration
- ADD/ADHD
- Trouble making decisions
- Poor memory
- Depression, irritability

- Mood disorders
- Pain and inflammation
- Immune system weakness
- Increased risk for heart disease, diabetes, cancer, and Alzheimer's
- Accelerated aging
- Weight gain

Insomnia is one of the most common complaints I hear from patients. This is what I recommend for getting a good night's sleep:

1. Set up a bedtime routine. Go to bed each night ideally by 10 PM, or at the very latest by 11. You feel so much more refreshed sleeping from 11 PM to 6 AM than from 1 AM to 8 AM. Wake up at the same time each morning. If you sleep in on the weekends, you may find it much harder to fall asleep early on Sunday night again.

2. Get outside each day for some fresh air and sunshine, even if it's just for a 15-minute walk at lunchtime. This can help increase nighttime melatonin production, which is a hormone vital for sleep.

3. Avoid using electronics one hour before bedtime. That includes computers, cell phones, tablets, and TV (especially the nightly news). It is too stimulating for your brain and can lower your melatonin production. You should use this time to relax, stretch, read, write in your journal, or plan your next day.

4. Have your last meal at least three hours before bedtime. However, if you tend to have low blood sugar, and you wake up each night at about 3 AM, have a light protein snack such as a handful of raw nuts or a small protein shake about 30 minutes before bed and see if that helps.

5. Drink most of your water earlier in the day and afternoon so that you can minimize water intake in the evening. This way you can prevent having to wake up in the middle of the night to go to the bathroom.

6. Magnesium works great for helping you relax and sleep better through the night. I usually recommend taking one to two Magnesium Malate capsules 30–60 minutes before bed.

7. If you suffer from pain, muscle tension, or headaches, this can certainly keep you from sleeping well.

One patient that comes to mind is a 40-year-old woman, named Doreen, who had chronic fatigue, inability to lose weight, migraine headaches, neck pain, jaw/TMJ pain, arm numbness and tingling, depression, anxiety, poor memory and concentration, dark circles under her eyes, digestive problems, and—you guessed it—insomnia. When she came in, she had a migraine for 16 days straight, despite all her medications and going to the hospital ER.

Besides doing lab testing and putting her on the FreeDiet® and Natural Medicine Formulas, I started treating her with gentle chiropractic adjustments, laser therapy, and myofascial release. Her migraine cleared up after one treatment and within one month, her neck pain, jaw pain, and arm numbness/tingling resolved, and she was sleeping through the night for the first time in years!

Seek the proper treatment if this is the case with you. It can help tremendously with sleep.

Chemical Stress

How do you avoid toxic chemicals in your environment? These can be a great source of stress to your system. Listed below are some ideas.

Oral Hygiene

Let's start with your mouth, as traditional toothpaste, mouthwash, and dental floss can have fluoride and other toxins. I would suggest a natural, fluoride-free toothpaste and dental floss. The same goes for mouthwash if you use one. Fluoride can interfere with iodine and have an adverse effect on thyroid function.

I recently saw a 50-year-old woman who had hyperthyroidism and was treated with radioactive iodine to destroy her thyroid before she saw me. One of the tests I ordered was a halides test, which checks iodine, bromine, and fluoride. Besides iodine deficiency, her fluoride levels were above optimal, as her city water contained fluoride. Although she had a water filter, it did not filter out fluoride, as this requires a special fluoride filter. She was also cooking with unfiltered water and was getting the full dose of fluoride there.

If you have fluoridated drinking water, I recommend investing in a water purification system that also filters out fluoride. See the Resources section in the back of this book for recommendations.

Facial Care

Use natural cleansers, shaving creams, acne products, and moisturizers to minimize your toxic chemical exposure in your facial care products. Many traditional products contain synthetic fragrances, petrochemicals, gluten, and other toxic ingredients.

Body Products

For soaps, bubble baths, and lotions, select natural products without gluten. Avoid aluminum containing deodorants and antiperspirants and opt for the natural ones instead. Many traditional body products are loaded with chemical toxins.

I had one patient with a 9 cm thyroid nodule and goiter who, on testing, was highly reactive to a chemical that was in body products. She worked in a cosmetics store and was in contact with their lotions and fragrances daily. Besides the FreeDiet®, getting out of that environment was one of the things that helped her recover and significantly shrink her nodule and goiter.

Hair Care

Traditional shampoos, conditioners, hair gels, hair sprays, and colorings can also have toxic chemicals. Choose natural products without gluten or synthetic fragrances.

Makeup

Traditional makeups can have toxic chemicals in them. I highly recommend using natural, gluten-free makeup products.

Nail Care

I recommend using nail polishes that are free of formaldehyde, toluene, and dibutyl phthalate and that are less toxic than the usual products.

Perfume and Cologne

I suggest using essential oil-based perfumes as opposed to the traditional, synthetic fragrances. You may not realize it, but synthetic fragrances can have many different toxic ingredients, including petrochemicals, and they don't have to disclose them on the label.

I had a patient years ago who would come in with the strongest smelling perfume. Within seconds of her entering the clinic, the smell would permeate the entire place. She was complaining about migraines—go figure! Upon my suggestion she stopped using the perfume and guess what happened? Her migraines went away! As a side benefit, we could all breathe a lot easier in our clinic.

Household Toxins

The tips below are many things you can do to clean up the chemicals in your house and minimize your toxic exposure.

Clean Water

It is very important to get a good water purifier. I recommend the Berkey Water Purifier for a countertop model or Aquasana Water Filter for under the sink. For a whole-house filter, I also recommend Aquasana as even with bathing and showering you can absorb chlorine and other toxins right through your skin. Instead of a whole house filter, they both have shower filters as well.

Kitchen

Avoid non-stick and aluminum cookware and instead use stainless steel, ceramic, or glass.

Using cast iron pans are fine if you are low in blood iron/ferritin levels but otherwise should be avoided. I treat many patients with high iron levels and cast-iron cookware is a common source of exposure.

I had a patient with high ferritin who swore she wasn't using cast-iron pans but upon further questioning it was discovered her grill grate that she barbecued with every night was cast iron. Porcelain coated cast iron or stainless steel are safer alternatives if you have high iron/ferritin blood levels.

Cleaning Agents

I recommend choosing natural window, counter, and floor cleaners and minimizing the use of chlorine and ammonia. You can use white vinegar, baking soda, and essential oils to make your own products, although there are many natural household products without synthetic fragrances on the market. This includes natural fragrance-free dish soap and dishwasher detergent as well.

Laundry

For laundry, I recommend using detergents that are free and clear of dyes, fragrances, and toxic chemicals. There are many brands on the market. The same goes for fabric softeners and dryer sheets. Traditional ones can be laden with toxic fragrances and chemicals.

Synthetic fragrances may contain numerous harmful ingredients, including carcinogenic chemicals, neurotoxins, respiratory irritants, solvents, aldehydes, petrochemicals, and phthalates, which can act as hormone disrupters.

Once, my wife, Dawn lent her sweater to someone, and when she got it back, they apparently laundered it using dryer strips. The smell was so strong we had to keep it in a plastic bag in the garage. The next day she put it through our washing machine and dryer. Still having a strong smell, she soaked it overnight and put it through the wash two more times. She still couldn't get out the smell. So much for that sweater.

Some of the most harmful ingredients in dryer sheets and liquid fabric softeners include benzyl acetate, benzyl alcohol, ethanol, and chloroform, which can be carcinogens, neurotoxins and/or respiratory tract irritants.

Another time, I was outside with my daughter, Adriana, who was about five years old at the time. She looked up and said, "Ew, what's that disgusting smell?!" It turns out that our neighbor was doing their laundry, and she could smell the strong synthetic fragrance of dryer strips in the air. Use natural alternatives!

For dry cleaning, do an internet search for non-toxic dry cleaners near you as they avoid using dangerous chemical solvents. Most cleaners us perchloroethylene, also known as perc which is reasonable considered to be a human carcinogen. High levels of residual perc have been found on dry-cleaned clothes.

Pest Control

Pesticides are another source of toxins. There are safer alternatives with products, including exterminators that use non-toxic methods.

Mold

Mold exposure is a common source of toxins. Chronic sinus issues, headaches, cough, asthma or other breathing difficulties, itchy eyes, fatigue, weakness, pain, diarrhea, lack of memory and concatenation, confusion, numbness, tingling, vertigo, and autoimmune conditions can all be related to mold exposure.

Air Fresheners and Candles

Use essential oils and avoid traditional air fresheners and synthetic fragrances. There are many essential oil diffusers on the market to choose from. You can also place some drops or essential oil in a glass spray bottle to freshen the room with.

An even better choice than candles would be to choose the battery-operated ones to keep the air clear. In the massage rooms at my prior clinic, the therapists burned natural, essential-oil candles with every massage. We thought that was okay, but after a couple of years the ceiling tiles and AC vents were covered with black soot. Imagine what you're breathing in!

Flame Retardants

A recent research study indicated that 80% of individuals tested had high levels of flame retardants in their blood. Polybrominated diphenyl ethers (PBDEs) were classified by the US EPA in 1995 as possible human carcinogens. They have been linked to many negative health effects including hormone disruption, liver damage, and impaired brain development in children. A major source of these is polyurethane foam, plastics, furniture, car seats, and mattresses. Children's costumes and some pajamas for infants also have flame retardants.

You can avoid these by choosing a mattress without chemical flame retardants and select a natural, organic latex mattress instead. There are many options out there, and I listed the bedding company we use for 100% natural, organic mattresses in the resource section in this book.

You can choose children's clothes without chemical flame retardants—100% cotton is best, especially organic. Due to increased awareness of this toxic issue, you can also look up car seat brands that don't use chemical flame retardants.

Clean Indoor Air

Air quality is so essential for our health. Common indoor pollutants include dust, pollen, pet dander, mold spores, smoke, VOCs from carpeting, building materials, paint, furniture, shower curtains, cleaning products, and fragrances.

Besides choosing natural alternatives when possible, you can let outside fresh air in if the conditions and air quality are right. Another solution is to use a high-quality air purifier that can remove all the above airborne toxins. Check the resource section for the type I most recommend.

Swimming Pools

Whether you have your own swimming pool or just use one, there are alternatives to traditional chlorine, like ionization, peroxide, and salt systems. If you do use chlorine, just make sure the levels are at one to three parts per million, as above that can be very toxic. You can easily test it yourself with some test strips you can buy online or at the local hardware store.

Even if you have a pool service, you should still test before swimming. We had our pool maintenance guy tell us after chlorine shocking the pool that it was safe for our daughter to swim in three hours. So, I kept checking the levels and it took two weeks to get down to three parts per million chlorine. It's best to test, not guess!

There would be times I would walk into a treatment room with a patient and the entire room would smell like chlorine. I would ask them if they were swimming recently, and they would say, "Oh, yes, I was swimming laps this morning." I thought so.

Years ago, my mother was visiting me and was in the hot tub at a local hotel. After 30 minutes, she came out and her blue-green bathing suit was bleached white! I suggest testing hotel/health club pools and hot tubs before using if you want to avoid excessive chlorine.

Chlorine being a halide can interfere with iodine and thus affect thyroid function. This is not good if you have hypothyroidism, thyroid nodules, or goiter.

Outdoors

If you're going to use sunscreen, use natural sunscreens that are free of synthetic fragrances.

There are also effective natural bug repellents that are free of toxic chemicals.

Regarding pesticides and weed killers, you want to avoid being outside when those are being used and avoid walking barefoot or playing on the grass for at least 48 hours afterward. This goes for your pets, too.

One time, my wife and I were at a charity event enjoying a nice evening with dozens of other guests on the pool patio of an exquisite home. Suddenly, the preprogrammed mosquito spray misters came on. Fortunately, we were able to quickly run inside before getting saturated with pesticides. Avoid exposure to toxic chemicals!

EMFs

Lastly, electromagnetic fields can be a great source of stress. Exposure to EMFs can increase free radical concentrations and result in oxidative stress in many tissues of the body. To lessen exposure, I suggest using your speakerphone as opposed to putting the cell phone to your ear, keeping it on airplane mode if you have it in your pocket, keeping it at least a few feet away from you while sleeping and preferably in the other room.

Sauna

Speaking of electromagnetic fields, a great way to detoxify your body is a low-EMF infrared sauna. I recommend doing this for 30-minute sessions two to three times per week. Preheat to 120 degrees Fahrenheit and turn up to 135 degrees upon going in. This is a great way to detoxify chemicals within your body, and it works great for pain and stress relief.

I found amazing benefits from doing this regularly. It feels like I just had both a massage and a workout after each session. This is one of the therapies we use at our Natural Medicine Clinic for eliminating high levels of toxic metals, including iron.

Those are some tips for identifying sources of toxins and stress in your home and alternatives for managing and reducing that stress and toxic load to your body.

Next, we're going to talk about how to achieve that next level of health: Functional & Free™!

CHAPTER 10

NEXT LEVEL HEALTH: FUNCTIONAL & FREE™

What is the next level of health beyond the FreeDiet®? Being Functional & Free™ is the ability to work, play, and function at your highest level. To be free of pain, fatigue, gut, thyroid, and other chronic health issues. To have vibrant energy, maintain your optimal weight, and feel the best you have in years!

Sometimes diet alone won't accomplish this, so we look in other areas to help you achieve vibrant health. Your health is largely dependent on three main areas—mental, physical, and chemical stress and how well you handle these.

When we look at chemical stress, we break that down into five categories—deficiencies, toxins, infections, hormones, and food reactions.

Deficiencies

Most of the patients I see are deficient in one or more nutrients, especially iron, vitamin B12, folate, vitamin D, magnesium, zinc, iodine, and selenium.

Some of this can be determined from regular blood tests but for a more comprehensive evaluation, I use a micronutrient panel that measures 38 different vitamins and minerals. This tests serum and white blood cell and red blood cell levels for a more thorough and accurate assessment.

For iodine testing, I recommend a urine test—both before and after an iodine loading dose and then a 24-hour urine collection. Another good option is a dried urine test upon arising and at bedtime.

There is a lot of controversy over iodine supplements. It seems that many doctors, health practitioners, and endocrinologists say that iodine is to be avoided by thyroid patients especially those with Hashimoto's and Graves' disease. While that may be true in some cases, that has not been my experience.

Most patients I test with thyroid autoimmune conditions, nodules, and/ or goiter have an iodine deficiency. The patients that I have helped shrink their thyroid nodules/goiter by over 30 percent in the first three months were all taking iodine based on their lab results.

These include patients with Hashimoto's that were taking 12.5 mg of iodine daily. I even had one patient with Graves' disease taking 12.5 mg iodine along with the FreeDiet® and other Natural Medicine Formulas, and her hyperthyroidism normalized in one month. This was with no medication, no surgery, and no radioactive iodine, all of which her endocrinologist told her were the only options.

Now I'm not suggesting you should start taking iodine. If you are deficient, it can be beneficial to supplement. Otherwise, I don't recommend taking a separate iodine supplement, as it could have adverse effects. I also recommend taking a selenium supplement and doing follow-up thyroid lab tests regularly—TSH, Free T4, Free T3, TPO and thyroglobulin Abs—while taking mg doses of iodine.

Toxins

A 33-year-old woman named Melanie came to see me who had symptoms of tremors, inner trembling, and shakiness with leg twitching at night in bed. She also had fatigue, brain fog, insomnia, eyelid twitching, bloating, gas, constipation, and diarrhea. Her primary doctor did some lab testing and recommended folic acid. She took folic acid daily and a bunch of other vitamin supplements with no improvement.

I ordered some comprehensive lab testing and one of the things that came back was extremely high levels of mercury in her blood. It turns out she was eating sushi multiple times a week, and the mercury from the fish accumulated in her body, causing her neurological symptoms. After doing the FreeDiet®, the appropriate Natural Medicine Formulas, and an oral chelating supplement for the excess mercury, her symptoms cleared up.

Besides heavy metal testing, if needed I check for non-metal toxins and mycotoxins (from toxic mold) through blood and or urine tests. Years ago, when I was feeling sick, I tested positive for arsenic. I wondered how it could be, as I was a vegetarian at the time, eating lots of healthy rice and vegetables while avoiding those "evil" meats. It turns out it was from all the rice consumption, including rice protein, which was in my detox shakes. Go figure—the most popular detox protein powder at the time was made with rice protein!

Speaking of metals, what about iron? Just as low iron can cause many symptoms, such as fatigue, brain fog, shortness of breath, heart palpitations, and hair loss, high iron levels can be even worse.

I had a 32-year-old patient named Sean who had fatigue, lack of focus and concentration, anxiety, lightheadedness, low libido, heart palpitations (PVCs), high blood pressure, and he was very thin. He had been to many different doctors and cardiologists to no avail. After I performed an evaluation and lab testing, I found his ferritin levels, which represent the amount of stored iron in your body, was at almost 600 ng/ml! Optimal levels are between 60 and 90.

After putting him on the FreeDiet® and our Natural Medicine Formulas, along with an oral chelating supplement and infrared sauna sessions, his levels dropped to 118 within two months, and all his symptoms cleared up. Even his high blood pressure was resolved.

The test for iron includes serum iron, TIBC, percent saturation, and ferritin levels. This is done in combination with a more complete panel which includes a CBC, chemistry panel, and other tests. The following is an example of one of the tests I run on most all our new patients.

Comprehensive Health Panel

- CMP (Comprehensive Metabolic Panel)
- CBC (Complete Blood Count) w/differential
- Lipid panel
- TSH (Thyroid Stimulating Hormone)
- T4, free
- T3, free
- Thyroglobulin antibodies
- TPO antibodies
- Reverse T3
- Iron, TIBC, percent saturation
- Ferritin
- LD (Lactate Dehydrogenase)
- Magnesium, RBC
- Uric acid
- Vitamin D, 25-OH
- Vitamin B12
- Folate
- DHEA sulfate
- Cortisol
- CRP, HS (C-Reactive Protein)
- Urinalysis
- IGF-1 (Insulin-Like Growth Factor 1—a growth hormone)
- SHBG (Sex Hormone Binding Globulin)
- Estradiol
- Testosterone, free
- Testosterone, total
- Progesterone (female)
- Homocysteine

Infections

You can follow the FreeDiet®, you can correct all your deficiencies, you can eliminate the toxins, but what happens if you have yeast or bacterial overgrowth in your gut? Or, God forbid, a parasite? I had all three of these at once. No wonder I was feeling so terrible!

I recommend comprehensive stool testing to find out and then treat it appropriately. The most common finding I see with my patients that have thyroid and digestive issues are yeast overgrowth, bacterial imbalance, H. pylori, and the parasite blastocystis hominis.

Then there are viruses that can be detected through blood testing. Epstein-Barr virus (EBV) is the most common virus that I see in our patients, especially those with autoimmune conditions such as Hashimoto's.

For all these findings, there are natural treatment protocols to help with healing. Refer to later chapters for more details on these.

Maintaining good oral hygiene is also essential. Periodontal infections have been linked to numerous adverse health effects that include diabetes, cardiovascular disease, respiratory infections, adverse pregnancy outcomes, rheumatoid arthritis, and Hashimoto's.

Hormones

It is important to look at each of these and have them in balance. Besides the Comprehensive Health Panel blood test above, I often order more in-depth hormone testing with urine or saliva to assess adrenal function. This is measured four times throughout the day to determine your daily fluctuation of adrenal hormones. This can pick up a deficiency or excess of adrenal hormones as well as estrogen, progesterone, testosterone, melatonin, and neurotransmitters.

Food sensitivities/allergies

There are two general methods to determine food sensitivities or allergies. One way is the elimination diet, and the second way is lab testing. A food allergy creates an almost immediate response, such as difficulty breathing, itchy throat, hives, abdominal pain, vomiting, or diarrhea. A food sensitivity is a delayed response. It could be a few hours to even up to a few days to see its effect, so it's harder to identify. That's why when we reintroduce new foods, it's at most one new food every three days.

Within the FreeDiet® is an elimination diet. After running countless food sensitivity and allergy tests over the last 33-plus years, there are certain foods that are most commonly reactive—gluten, grains, sugar, yeast, dairy, eggs, soy, legumes, nightshades—and those are many of the foods in the avoid section of FreeDiet® Phase 1.

Sometimes, however, you can be allergic or sensitive to seemingly healthy foods. For instance, I have, on rare occasions, had patients test positive for allergies or sensitivities to lemon, avocado, flax, coconut, or psyllium. Most people do extremely well on the FreeDiet®, and if there are still some lingering symptoms, lab testing can help identify these hidden food sensitivities.

I had a patient with chronic migraines which cleared up on the FreeDiet®. Whenever she would get exposed inadvertently to gluten, she would get a headache. One time she was eating out and by the time she got home, she had a headache. When she called and spoke to the chef, it turns out that there was lemon on the fish. That's one of the foods that she tested positive for.

If food allergies are suspected, I recommend an IgE blood test for at least 25 foods. I will sometimes run a 96-food IgE panel if I suspect allergies to be a significant issue.

For food sensitivities, I prefer a profile that tests for multiple types of delayed sensitivity reactions, which can be more accurate and reliable than only IgG antibodies and other single types of food sensitivity testing. This is based on using many different labs for my own testing and for numerous patients over the past 33-plus years.

Gluten Sensitivity/Celiac/Intestinal Permeability

Gluten has its own category amongst foods because gluten sensitivity is so widespread and can have such devastating effects. It is the most common food sensitivity I see, and most of my patients test positive for this.

It's important to realize that only about 50 percent of people with gluten sensitivity or celiac disease have digestive complaints.

The main difference between non-celiac gluten sensitivity (NCGS) and celiac disease is that celiac is a genetic autoimmune disorder that involves intestinal damage from gluten, but otherwise the symptoms of both conditions are similar. The list of symptoms is vast and includes over 200 symptoms and conditions.

I had a patient, a 74-year-old woman, whose major complaint was chronic knee pain due to arthritis. After testing positive for gluten sensitivity and starting the FreeDiet®, which of course is free of gluten and grains, her knee pain cleared up. Whenever she would eat anything with gluten, her knee pain would return by the next day.

In some people, neurological effects are the main symptoms, including numbness and tingling, anxiety, depression, bipolar, and brain fog. I had a 42-year-old patient, Jeanne, who tested positive for gluten sensitivity and improved so much on the FreeDiet® that she was able to get off the antidepressant medication she had been on for years. Oh, and she lost 50 pounds in six months.

How do you test for gluten sensitivity? I do not recommend the standard celiac or gluten sensitivity test that you can get at the major labs through your doctor, as they only measure one to five different antibodies as opposed to the 30 to 40 that are available. There are many false negatives, and people are thinking they're fine with gluten when they're not.

I use and recommend a comprehensive wheat gluten/celiac panel, which measures 40 different antibodies to gluten, gliadins, non-gluten wheat proteins, wheat allergy, celiac antibodies, and celiac genetic markers.

This test also measures intestinal permeability, also known as leaky gut. This is important information to know, as leaky gut can lead to autoimmune conditions, digestive issues, skin reactions, joint pain, and a whole host of symptoms. The good news is that it can be healed. I have helped many patients using a three-month protocol with Natural Medicine Formulas and the FreeDiet® to help heal leaky gut.

In general, if any of your chronic symptoms persist after doing the FreeDiet®, then I suggest you see a Functional Medicine practitioner near you for evaluation and testing. The following is the proprietary process I use with patients at the Natural Medicine Clinic.

Functional & Free™

A 5-Step Program to determine your root cause and provide you with whole-body, permanent solutions.

1. *Whole-body health analysis to determine the root cause of your condition.*
   - Spend time listening to your story and what your health goals are.
   - Review of your medical history and current symptoms.
   - Physical evaluation (if in person) including vital signs, orthopedic, neuromuscular, and postural assessments.
   - Determine which lab tests or other diagnostic tests are necessary and interpret the results.
   - Evaluate your findings and thoroughly analyze your lab results to determine the root cause of your condition.

2. *Permanent Solutions: reveal the root cause of your condition and provide clear solutions for you to get better.*
   - Review your evaluation and lab findings with you.
   - Go over in detail your nutrition plan, including specific supplement recommendations.
   - Review your treatment plan, including recommended follow-up visits and testing to ensure you are making progress and getting the results you're looking for.

3. *The FreeDiet®*

A proprietary diet that's free of the most common allergens and sensitivities so that you can identify and eliminate the foods most responsible for pain, gut and thyroid issues, autoimmune and other chronic health conditions. It's a diet that reduces inflammation and promotes healthy digestion, vibrant energy, and the ability to fit into clothes you haven't worn in years.

4. *Natural Medicine Formulas®*

A therapeutic, professional line of supplements that support your digestive and immune health and balance your system to give you more energy and mental clarity.

5. *"Free for Life": continue to have your body work the way it's supposed to work so that you're free to live the way you want to live.*
   • Receive accountability and check-ins with the doctor and our team.
   • Follow up testing as needed with changes to your diet and supplements.
   • Receive guidance on lifestyle habits, such as exercise, stress relief, proper sleep, and minimizing toxins to continue your journey toward lifelong vibrant health.

And if someone has a structural issue which needs manual treatment and therapies:

6. *"Healing Hands" to relieve pain, improve function, and get you feeling the best you have in years.*
   • Soft tissue neuromuscular therapy, which includes myofascial release and trigger point therapy, to reduce myofascial trigger points, adhesions, and fibrous tissue for quick pain relief.
   • Gentle chiropractic adjustments (no cracking) with the Impulse instrument to relieve pain and restore normal joint function and movement.
   • Super Pulsed Laser Therapy to reduce pain and inflammation and enhance microcirculation to promote healing.

7. *Functional Fitness Training*

Specific Exercises to improve strength, flexibility, balance, and posture, and to ensure that your improvements are long-lasting.

I believe that any health problem has a solution. Find the root cause of the problem, and you can find the solution!

The following chapters include information on eight of the most common conditions that I've helped patients improve or resolve. Read the ones that are most suited to you.

CHAPTER 11

THE FREEDIET® FIX FOR THYROID NODULES

We get so many people contacting us from around the world for help with their thyroid nodules and/or goiter. The most common story I hear is that their doctors tell them after the ultrasound that they need a needle biopsy. After the biopsy, they are told the only way to address these larger nodules is to have surgery.

For some, the thought of getting needles stuck in their neck is not very comforting, and certainly surgery in that area with the possible long-term side effects is scary for most. Then they would depend on lifelong medications without even figuring out what caused the nodules in the first place.

They're told there is no other option and that surgery is the only answer once these nodules get to a certain size, even though more than 95 percent of these are benign (noncancerous).

I have found that there are other solutions to shrinking thyroid nodules. Although I had treated thousands of patients with thyroid disorders and Hashimoto's, my focus wasn't on shrinking thyroid nodules—until one morning when my wife, Dawn, woke up with a bulge in her neck. We had an ultrasound done and found she had multiple nodules. One of them was 2.1 cm, so her doctor wanted her to do a needle biopsy, which my wife was petrified of.

Her doctor agreed to check it again in three months, and Dawn sought my help with this. I put her on the FreeDiet® and our Natural Medicine Formulas based on her lab results, and she noticed a significant improvement within two weeks. On the follow-up ultrasound at seven weeks, her nodule had shrunk by over 50 percent! She was very happy that her doctor said she no longer needed to get the biopsy done.

After helping many patients shrink their thyroid nodules, there are some general patterns I've noticed. Of course, I recommend getting an evaluation and proper lab testing to determine specifically what's going on. I do realize that some are not in a location or position to be able to do that. In that case, what I've generally found is:

Deficiencies

Iodine is almost always deficient in patients I see with nodules. This is not surprising, as years ago it was recognized as a primary cause of goiter. As a matter of fact, in the United States, the Midwest was referred to as the "Goiter Belt" because of the rampant iodine deficiencies in the middle of the country and the increased prevalence of goiter that developed. Federal law then mandated that iodine be added to salt, which helped reduce the incidence of goiter.

Now that seems to have been forgotten because iodine is rarely ever mentioned or tested for in patients that have thyroid nodules or goiter. It is quite the opposite. Most doctors and endocrinologists recommend avoiding iodine like the plague. Having surgery they think is okay, though.

The test I run on patients is a first-morning urine iodine test, followed by a 50 mg loading dose of iodine and then collecting the urine for 24 hours. Most patients test low on both. Another testing option is a dried urine collection first thing in the morning and then at bedtime.

If you are deficient in iodine, it can be very helpful to supplement. Otherwise, I don't recommend taking a separate iodine supplement. I also recommend follow-up thyroid lab tests regularly while taking mg doses of iodine, as well as taking selenium.

One patient, a 60-year-old woman named Cindy, drove two and a half hours to see me because of her multinodular goiter including a 9 cm nodule. She was so uncomfortable and embarrassed by it and was told she had to get surgery. Testing revealed she was deficient in iodine, so I had her taking 12.5 mg per day. She also used 200 mcg of selenium with this, which is very important when taking iodine.

After three months on the FreeDiet® and Natural Medicine Formulas, including iodine, an ultrasound revealed her thyroid nodules and goiter shrunk by an average of 33 percent. She also cleared up her digestive issues, fatigue, brain fog, insomnia, and headaches.

Vitamin D deficiency is another common thing I see with thyroid patients. The most common dose I recommend is 5000 IU with vitamin K2, and testing can determine this more specifically.

In general, I recommend:

The Functional Five supplements:
- ActivMulti™ without Iron—multivitamin
- OmegaSorb 3X™—fish oil
- D3 5000 + K2
- Magnesium Malate (Magnesium Citrate if have constipation)
- ProbioSupreme™30—probiotics

- Iodine Protect™ (if deficient)—potassium iodide and iodine
- Selenium (selenomethionine)
- MethylFolate B12 Plus—methylfolate with B12
- Iron Glycinate (if ferritin is less than 50 ng/ml)
- Zinc Glycinate
- C-Bioflavonoids 500—vitamin C with bioflavonoids
- GastricZyme™—betaine HCL with pepsin and gentian
- NAC (N-Acetyl Cysteine)

Toxins

Most of my patients with nodules and/or goiter have toxins show up in their blood or urine. Cindy had a positive immune reaction to a chemical that she was exposed to daily, as she worked in a cosmetics store.

I recommend the FreeDiet® 3-Minute Super Smoothie, as it is very nourishing and very cleansing. I also recommend infrared sauna therapy, as this helps sweat out many different toxins.

This patient had high iron and ferritin levels, so if that is the case you would avoid iron. The infrared sauna can be especially helpful for iron overload.

Hormones

Besides thyroid hormone imbalances, hormonal deficiencies or excess, including estrogen, progesterone, and testosterone, are very common. Also, common findings are adrenal hormones—high or low cortisol and DHEA. This can demonstrate the effects stress has on your thyroid and health in general.

Infections

The most common infections I see with patients that have thyroid nodules are yeast overgrowth, bacterial overgrowth, and/or parasites, based on stool test results. Epstein-Barr virus is also common.

For these I recommend:
- Yeast Defeat™
- Microb-Balance™
- ImmunoSilver™—silver solution
- Monolaurin
- Gut Immune Repair™ DF

Food Reactions

This is where the FreeDiet® is so helpful, as you are avoiding the most commonly reactive foods that can be responsible for inflammation and thyroid issues.

Sometimes from doing food sensitivity lab testing, I will see foods that are not in Phase 1, so that certainly can be useful to know. I've seen reactions to foods like turkey, lemon, cashews, and coconut. These are rare, but it could be helpful to get tested if someone wasn't quite getting the expected results.

It's usually not just a single cause but many factors that are involved. This was the case with Janelle, a 36-year-old woman, who was told she needed surgery for her 4-plus cm thyroid nodule. Not wanting to go under the knife, she came to see me and was able to shrink her nodule by 73 percent, as well as resolve her fatigue, brain fog, headaches, digestive issues, and weight loss resistance after three months on the FreeDiet®. During this time, she dropped 23 pounds!

The following factors normalized after the initial four weeks on the FreeDiet®: high CRP inflammatory marker, high ferritin, high DHEA, high testosterone, high estrogen, and low progesterone. Other root causes were a deficiency in iodine and other nutrients, excess fluoride, gluten, yeast and other food sensitivities, dysbiosis (imbalanced microbiome), and leaky gut.

It's important to realize that thyroid nodules are a response to something wrong in the body. I believe that if you can find out what the underlying causes are, then you can come up with a solution on how to fix them. You didn't always have thyroid nodules. At some point, you had a healthy thyroid, and then suddenly or over time, you developed these nodules. What caused this inflammation and swelling? It's the result of these five main things: deficiencies, toxins, infections, hormones, and food reactions.

You can get better. You just need to find out what's causing it and apply those solutions.

CHAPTER 12

THE FREEDIET® FIX FOR HASHIMOTO'S AND AUTOIMMUNE CONDITIONS

This is a subject near and dear to me, as years ago I was diagnosed with the thyroid autoimmune condition called Hashimoto's as well as rheumatoid arthritis. This was an important part in the evolution of the FreeDiet®, as I had to figure out a way to get better. I was able to resolve these conditions, with my antibodies being in the normal range for the past 10-plus years.

These are the common things I find in the many patients I've helped reverse Hashimoto's and other autoimmune conditions:

Deficiencies

In general, I recommend:

The Functional Five:
- ActivMulti™ without Iron—multivitamin
- OmegaSorb 3X™—fish oil
- D3 5000 + K2
- Magnesium Malate (Magnesium Citrate if have constipation)
- ProbioSupreme™30—probiotics

- Iodine Protect™ (if deficient)—potassium iodide and iodine
- Selenium (selenomethionine)
- MethylFolate B12 Plus—methylfolate with B12
- Iron Glycinate (if ferritin is less than 50 ng/ml)
- Zinc Glycinate

- C-Bioflavonoids 500—vitamin C with bioflavonoids
- GastricZyme™—betaine HCL with pepsin and gentian
- NAC (N-Acetyl Cysteine)
- Curcumin Protect™—high absorption curcumin supplement
- Inositol (Myo and D-chiro)

For iodine deficiency, it can be very helpful to supplement. Otherwise, I don't recommend taking a separate iodine supplement, as it could be counterproductive. I also recommend follow-up thyroid lab tests regularly while taking mg doses of iodine.

Toxins

I usually see heavy metals, fluoride, or iron overload. For which I recommend:

- Infrared sauna
- NAC (N-Acetyl Cysteine)
- Metal Cleanse™—oral chelating formula

Infections

After testing patients, I almost always find yeast overgrowth, bacterial overgrowth including H. Pylori, and/or parasites. The body is mounting an attack against these critters and ultimately starts destroying your own tissue, such as thyroid in Hashimoto's, joints in rheumatoid arthritis, or nervous system in multiple sclerosis. Epstein-Barr virus is a common finding as well.

Recommended supplements:

- Yeast Defeat™
- Microb-Balance™
- ImmunoSilver™—silver solution
- ProbioSupreme™ Sb
- Monolaurin

Leaky gut is a common cause/trigger for autoimmune conditions. In addition to the FreeDiet®, I recommend a three-month supplement protocol to help heal leaky gut.

- GI-Mend™—gut support formula
- ProbioXtreme™350—probiotic
- Gut Immune Repair™—immunoglobulin concentrate
- FreeDiet™ Protein—high in collagen

Food reactions

Gluten is a huge factor in Hashimoto's and autoimmune conditions. The FreeDiet® is a truly gluten-free diet that is free of gluten, grains, sugar, yeast, dairy, eggs, soy, legumes, nightshades, and processed foods. These are the foods most commonly responsible for autoimmune, digestive issues, and other chronic health conditions.

I had a patient, a 54-year-old woman, whose thyroglobulin antibody levels were 5475 IU/ml (normal <40) as well as TPO of 272 IU/ml (normal <35). She was able to get down to normal over a period of two years on the FreeDiet® and Natural Medicine Formulas. As with most Hashimoto's patients, she had many things going on, including deficiencies, toxins, hormonal imbalance, infections—yeast, parasites, and bacterial overgrowth—and food reactions.

Most of the foods you would typically react to are eliminated with FreeDiet® Phase 1. If you found your antibody levels still weren't declining, then you could get tested and see what other foods you are reacting to, or if there are deficiencies, toxins, hormonal issues, or infections lurking.

CHAPTER 13

THE FREEDIET® FIX FOR DIGESTIVE ISSUES: IBS AND PARASITES

O f all the new patients that come in to see me with all the different health conditions, the most common underlying theme is digestive symptoms. This includes bloating, gas, abdominal pain, indigestion, reflux, heartburn, IBS, IBD, colitis, diarrhea, and/or constipation. The FreeDiet® works amazingly well for these, as it eliminates the foods most commonly responsible for chronic digestive issues and inflammation.

There are other factors besides diet, however, that are sometimes involved. I recommend for my patients with digestive symptoms to get the proper lab testing to rule out the overgrowth of bacteria, yeast, and parasites. I had chronic digestive complaints for many years, including abdominal pain, indigestion, gas, bloating, and diarrhea. I was shocked to see my stool test results indicate yeast and bacterial overgrowth, as well as a parasite called blastocystis hominis.

After 13 years of trying many different natural products, supplements, herbs, remedies, and even prescription drugs, I finally figured out a protocol that worked. Then it took me less than six months to wipe it out. I never would have figured it out if I didn't get the initial stool test and then regular follow-up testing to make sure it was gone. Test, don't guess!

If you are not able to get specific testing, there are some general recommendations and findings I see with these patients that can help.

The Functional Five:

- ActivMulti™ without Iron—multivitamin
- OmegaSorb 3X™—fish oil
- D3 5000 + K2
- Magnesium Malate (Magnesium Citrate if have constipation)
- ProbioSupreme™30—probiotics

Deficiencies

Most commonly digestive enzymes are deficient, in which case I recommend:

- GastricZyme™—betaine HCL with pepsin and gentian root
- Zinc Glycinate

Toxins

Choose organic as much as possible, as pesticides and GMO foods are best to be avoided.

Infections—Bacterial overgrowth, yeast, parasites

- Yeast Defeat™
- Microb-Balance™
- ImmunoSilver™—silver solution
- ProbioSupreme™ Sb
- Appropriate homeopathic formulas

Leaky Gut

- GI-Mend™— gut support formula
- ProbioXtreme™350—high potency probiotic
- Curcumin Protect™—high absorption curcumin
- FreeDiet™ Protein or Paleo Protein—an excellent source of collagen
- Gut Immune Repair™ DF

Food Sensitivities

As far as food sensitivities go, the FreeDiet® eliminates the most common food reactions. If you're still having any digestive symptoms after completing the FreeDiet® Phase 1, then you can do food allergy and food sensitivity testing, which can further clarify if any other foods that are problematic.

I had a patient that was doing so much better in all areas, but she was still getting bloated after meals. After food sensitivity testing, it turned out one of the foods she was sensitive to was coconut, of all things. After removing this from her diet, her bloating cleared up.

Often, digestive issues lead to other symptoms as well. A 57-year-old patient I saw with reflux was diagnosed with GERD and Barrett's esophagus. His doctor prescribed acid-blocking medication and said he had to take it the rest of his life as there was no cure. Not wanting to do this, he contacted me for help. After an evaluation and testing, he started the FreeDiet® and Natural Medicine Formulas® and his reflux symptoms cleared up within a month.

A year later, his follow up endoscopy showed no signs of Barrett's esophagus! His doctor was quite surprised and said, "whatever voodoo you're doing, keep it up." What also cleared up was his fatigue, brain fog, skin problems, and chronic hip pain.

Heal your gut, and you can heal the rest of your body.

CHAPTER 14

THE FREEDIET® FIX FOR PAIN

D o you have pain you're dealing with that you would like to get rid of? It could be headaches, neck or back pain, joint pain, TMJ, numbness and tingling, or muscle aches. In this chapter, I'll review some common causes and solutions to help you resolve your pain.

If you are in pain, it can make you irritable, moody, depressed, and unable to concentrate. Pain can make you tense and keep you from sleeping well through the night. Pain can make you tired and adversely affect every area of your life.

Common medical treatments don't offer any real solutions. For instance, WebMD, the number one "health" website has this advice for pain treatment: a choice of five pain relievers, eight different antidepressants, five anticonvulsants (originally developed for epilepsy), or three different opioid painkillers, such as codeine, morphine, or oxycodone. And painkillers are the most common cause of drug addictions and drug overdose deaths in the United States.

I call them accidental drug addicts. They don't choose to use illicit narcotics; they're prescribed painkillers for an injury or post-surgical pain, and they soon became addicted. When they can't get any more, heroin is how they get their fix. Many lives have been ruined or abruptly ended.

Besides all the side effects and dependency with the above drugs, they do nothing to resolve the cause of the pain. How about getting to the root cause, and then you can have some permanent solutions.

What causes pain? Quite simply, let's break it down into three broad categories of chemical, physical, and mental stress.

Chemical stress

Food Sensitivities

Food reactions are a common cause of pain. The FreeDiet® can help dramatically with this, as it eliminates those foods—gluten, grains, sugar, yeast, dairy, eggs, soy, legumes, nightshades, and processed foods—most commonly responsible for inflammation.

I had a 58-year-old patient who had migraines and neck pain for many years. She was missing a lot of work and was on many different medications. She went on the FreeDiet® and was getting treatment, and her migraines cleared up. Her regular headaches, which she was getting very often, and her migraines both cleared up within one month, and she'd had these for years.

As long as she avoided her most sensitive foods, which were gluten and yeast, her headaches stayed away. As soon as she would accidentally or on purpose eat something containing these, her headaches would come roaring back.

I had another patient, Anthony, who was 57 years old and had chronic hip pain. His doctor prescribed medication but had no solutions. After doing the FreeDiet®, his hip pain completely resolved. What he discovered after this is that whenever he would eat gluten, his hip pain would come back within 24 hours. So now he doesn't eat gluten.

Deficiencies

Common causes of pain, headaches, numbness, and tingling that I see with patients are deficiencies in:
- Magnesium
- Vitamin D
- Vitamin B12
- Iron

Magnesium deficiency can cause muscle aches and stiffness, headaches, numbness, and tingling. I've had patients with chronic pain for years have it cleared up by testing and then giving the proper dosage of vitamin D. Among many other symptoms, vitamin B12 deficiency can cause numbness, tingling, and muscle weakness.

I've had patients with iron deficiency who have headaches, chest pain, and restless legs. I've seen these symptoms resolve when the deficiencies were corrected.

Other supplements that can help are curcumin and fish oil supplements, which help support a normal inflammatory response.

If thyroid hormones are low, that can contribute to pain, numbness, tingling, and headaches.

The same with low adrenal function, which can contribute to pain and inflammation.

The Functional Five supplements are recommended:
- ActivMulti™ without Iron—multivitamin
- OmegaSorb 3X™—fish oil
- D3 5000 + K2
- Magnesium Malate (Magnesium Citrate if have constipation)
- ProbioSupreme™30—probiotics

And depending on lab test findings:
- B12 Supreme™—sublingual methylcobalamin 5000 mcg
- Iron Glycinate (if ferritin is less than 50 ng/ml)
- C-Bioflavonoids 500—vitamin C with bioflavonoids
- Curcumin Protect™—high absorption curcumin supplement
- DHEA (if serum levels are below 100 and other factors)
- Cortisol Quencher™—adrenal support if cortisol is too high
- Adrenal Vibrance™—adrenal support if cortisol is too low
- T3 Balance™ and/or other thyroid support formulas (based on testing)

Toxins

Mercury, arsenic, or iron overload are common findings and can contribute to pain, numbness, tingling, and headaches.

Recommended supplements:
- NAC (N-Acetyl Cysteine)
- Metal Cleanse™—oral chelating formula
- Infrared sauna therapy 30 minutes two to three times per week at 120–135 degrees Fahrenheit.

Infections

Yeast, bacterial overgrowth, and/or parasites in the intestines, as well as Epstein-Barr virus are common causes of pain.

For these I recommend:
- Yeast Defeat™
- Microb-Balance™
- ImmunoSilver™—silver solution
- Vit C-Bioflavonoids 500—vitamin C with bioflavonoids
- Monolaurin

Leaky gut is often involved, as bacterial or yeast overgrowth and gluten sensitivities are a common cause. Increased intestinal permeability can contribute to systemic inflammation and pain.

Additional supplements I recommend for this are:
- GI-Mend™—gut support formula
- ProbioXtreme™350—high potency probiotic
- Gut Immune Repair™—immunoglobulin concentrate

Physical Stress

Myofascial trigger points are one of the most common causes of persistent pain. Trigger points are tender, tight bands or "knots" within a muscle that can also refer pain to other areas of the body. They can become fibrous and hard over time.

This can be referred to as myofascial pain, and you can have multiple trigger points throughout your body. For instance, trigger points in your neck and jaw can cause headaches and TMJ pain, trigger points in your low back and buttocks can cause sciatica, and trigger points in your calves and feet can cause foot and heel pain. Myofascial trigger points or muscular adhesions can also cause nerve entrapment, leading to numbness and tingling in your arms or legs.

These trigger points can be caused by an accident or injury, even one from years prior. Myofascial pain can also be caused gradually from repetitive stress, by doing the same type of activities over and over again. Things like sports, sitting at a computer, or using your smartphone for hours a day.

Even though myofascial trigger points are one of the most common causes of pain, they cannot be identified on x-ray or MRI. This leads many doctors to think that your pain is not real and is due to stress or is all in your head.

Another cause of persistent pain is joint dysfunction. This is where the joints of your spine or extremities can become stiff, stuck, or fixated, and they don't have normal motion. This can cause local pain and inflammation, irritate nerves, and can result in headaches, neck or back pain, TMJ, shoulder, knee, hip, or other joint pain.

How to eliminate structural/physical causes of pain:

1. Soft tissue treatments, such as Active Release Technique, which is a type of myofascial release or manual therapy, to reduce pain-producing myofascial trigger points, adhesions, and fibrous tissue, and to restore muscular balance.

2. Gentle chiropractic adjustments to restore normal joint function and movement. Instead of manual manipulation (cracking your neck or back), I prefer to use a computerized instrument called the Impulse. This is a very advanced, gentle, and precise way to reduce pain and restore motion to joints.

3. Super Pulsed Laser Therapy to reduce pain and inflammation and enhance microcirculation to promote healing.

4. Therapeutic functional training exercises to improve strength, flexibility, balance, and posture.

Mental/Emotional Stress

Stress can increase muscle tension, which decreases blood flow and increases pain. People have different areas of weakness that their mental stress seems to settle in. For some, it's the shoulders and neck, for others the jaw, and another common area is the low back. Pain anywhere in the body can be triggered by stress.

Stress-relieving techniques that can help reduce this aspect of pain:
Exercise
Prayer
Meditation
Massage
Spending time with nature
Getting outside for some sunshine
Recreation

Spending time with loved ones

Laughing

Having fun

Going on vacation

Getting enough sleep

Changing your focus is helpful as well. Many people keep themselves in a state of anxiety and pain because they are spending many hours per day on the internet asking, "What's wrong with me?" or "Why do I feel so bad?"

Instead ask, "How can I get better?" or "Who can I seek out for guidance to help me regain my health?" or "How can I find out what is causing this and take the action steps to get well?"

I don't find that mental stress alone is a cause of pain but certainly a contributing factor. Chronic pain can get better and often requires a multifaceted approach. Many get better with the FreeDiet® alone. Others need to delve further and address other underlying root causes. I believe if you find the root cause, you can be provided with long-term permanent solutions, and you can get better.

CHAPTER 15

THE FREEDIET® FIX FOR FATIGUE AND BRAIN FOG

Another common symptom for new patients is fatigue, whether it's difficulty getting out of bed in the morning, being sleepy in the afternoon, or just tired all day long. Brain fog usually goes along with this, which is basically fatigue of your brain. This includes a lack of focus and concentration, loss of memory, ADD, and ADHD. You're just not as sharp as you used to be, and you don't want to end up like your mother or grandmother, who had dementia.

You go to your doctor and they ask: How long have you been tired?

You: Oh, two or three years.

Doctor: Okay, well, then you have chronic fatigue syndrome.

You: What's that?

Doctor: That's when you're tired for a long time. We don't really know what causes it.

You: Are there any tests for it?

Doctor: Well...no.

You: Then how do I fix it?

Doctor: There is no known cure. You can take these antidepressants and ADHD drugs, that may help.

That's certainly one way to go—choose medicine. But if you want to get to the underlying root cause and *choose health*, these are the most common things I find:

Deficiencies:

- Iron
- Vitamin B12
- Folate
- Magnesium
- Vitamin D

The Functional Five are recommended:

ActivMulti™ without Iron—multivitamin
- OmegaSorb 3X™—fish oil
- D3 5000 + K2
- Magnesium Malate (Magnesium Citrate if have constipation)
- ProbioSupreme™30—probiotics

And depending on lab test findings:

- B12 Supreme™—sublingual methylcobalamin 5000 mcg
- MethylFolate B12 Plus—methylfolate with B12
- Iron Glycinate
- Iodine Protect™ (if deficient)—potassium iodide and iodine
- Selenium (selenomethionine)
- Iron Glycinate (if ferritin is less than 50 ng/ml)
- Zinc Glycinate
- C-Bioflavonoids 500—vitamin C with bioflavonoids
- GastricZyme™—betaine HCL with pepsin and gentian
- Curcumin Protect™—high absorption curcumin supplement
- DHEA (if serum levels are below 100 and other factors)
- Cortisol Quencher™—adrenal support if cortisol is too high
- Adrenal Vibrance™—adrenal support if cortisol is too low
- T3 Balance™ and/or other thyroid support formulas (based on testing)

Toxins

Mercury, arsenic, and/or iron overloads are common findings.

Recommended supplements:
- N-Acetyl Cysteine (NAC)
- Metal Cleanse™—oral chelating formula
- Infrared sauna therapy 30 minutes two to three times per week at 120–135 degrees Fahrenheit.

Infections

Yeast and/or bacterial overgrowth in the intestines, parasites, and/or Epstein-Barr virus are common causes of fatigue and brain fog.

For this I recommend:
- Yeast Defeat™
- Microb-Balance™
- ImmunoSilver™—silver solution
- C-Bioflavonoids 500—vitamin C with bioflavonoids
- Monolaurin

Leaky gut is often involved, as bacterial or yeast overgrowth and gluten sensitivities are a common cause. Increased intestinal permeability can contribute to both fatigue and brain fog.

Additional supplements I recommend for this are:
- GI-Mend™—gut support formula
- ProbioXtreme™ 350—high potency probiotic
- Gut Immune Repair™—immunoglobulin concentrate

Food Sensitivities

Food reactions are a common cause of fatigue and brain fog. The FreeDiet® can help dramatically with these. If you are still having significant symptoms after FreeDiet® Phase 1, then you may be still eating foods that you're sensitive to. This is a big source of fatigue, so food sensitivity and/or allergy testing may be recommended.

I saw a 43-year-old woman named Shari who was experiencing severe fatigue, chronic pain, insomnia, brain fog, dizziness, headaches, IBS, anxiety, and depression—all the typical chronic fatigue/fibromyalgia symptoms. Her doctor ran lab tests and said there was nothing wrong. He said, "Well, you have four kids, no wonder you're tired!" Of course, there was no shortage of drugs he prescribed.

I did an evaluation with comprehensive lab testing. Shari had anemia due to a severe iron deficiency. Her ferritin level, which can represent stored iron, was only 7 ng/ml, whereas the optimal range is 60–90. She was also deficient in vitamin D, magnesium, and vitamin B12. No wonder she was feeling so miserable.

After the first month of following the FreeDiet® and taking Natural Medicine Formulas to correct her deficiencies, her symptoms dramatically improved and she felt like she got her life back, the best she felt in years! She was even able to keep the four kids.

CHAPTER 16

THE FREEDIET® FIX FOR FAT

A 35-year-old woman named Beth came in with the usual symptoms of pain, fatigue, headaches, brain fog, sinus congestion, PMS, abdominal pain, bloating, and constipation. She was also unable to lose weight. She went on many different diets with no results. She even did the keto diet and lost only two or three pounds in a month's time, while running and weightlifting six times per week! After some lab testing, I put her on the FreeDiet®. In the first two weeks, she dropped ten pounds, and most of her symptoms had cleared up.

When losing or gaining weight, it's not all about the calories, per se. Food sensitivities are a huge part of the inability to lose weight. Even with keto, if you're eating foods you're sensitive or allergic to, you may have a hard time losing weight.

Hormones

Additional factors with weight loss under hormones are, first and foremost, thyroid. Many new patients come in and say they had their thyroid checked and the doctor said it's fine—but their doctor did not run the complete testing, just one or two thyroid numbers. You want to get comprehensive lab work, which includes six different thyroid values—TSH, Free T3, Free T4, Thyroglobulin antibodies, TPO antibodies, and reverse T3. Balancing your thyroid is very important for metabolism and weight loss.

Adrenal hormones (cortisol, DHEA-S), estrogen, progesterone, and testosterone are also important to assess, as are other factors. See Chapter 10 for details on lab testing.

Deficiencies

Common deficiencies I see are vitamin D, iron, vitamin B12, magnesium, and zinc. These can all affect your metabolism and ability to lose weight.

The Functional Five are recommended:
- ActivMulti™ without Iron—multivitamin
- OmegaSorb 3X™—fish oil
- D3 5000 + K2
- Magnesium Malate (Magnesium Citrate if have constipation)
- ProbioSupreme™30—probiotics

And depending on lab test findings:
- B12 Supreme™—sublingual methylcobalamin 5000 mcg
- MethylFolate B12 Plus—methylfolate with B12
- Zinc Glycinate
- C-Bioflavonoids 500—vitamin C with bioflavonoids
- Curcumin Protect™—high absorption curcumin supplement
- DHEA (if serum levels are below 100 and other factors)
- Cortisol Quencher™—if cortisol is too high
- Fem Synergy™—for hormone support
- Thyroid support (based on testing)

Toxins

High levels of heavy metals like mercury, arsenic, lead, iron, or petro-chemicals can affect your ability to lose weight.

Recommended supplements:
- N-Acetyl Cysteine (NAC)
- Metal Cleanse™—oral chelating formula

Infrared sauna therapy 30 minutes two to three times per week at 120–135 degrees Fahrenheit.

Infections

Yeast and/or bacterial overgrowth in the intestines, parasites, and/or Epstein-Barr virus can all affect your metabolism.

Depending on your findings, I recommend:
- Yeast Defeat™
- Microb-Balance™
- ImmunoSilver™—silver solution
- Gut Immune Repair™ DF
- Monolaurin

Food Reactions

Eating foods that you're sensitive or allergic to can affect your ability to lose weight, which is one reason why the FreeDiet® is so effective. In FreeDiet® Phase 2, when you're adding foods back one at a time, one of the signs of food sensitivity is gaining two or more pounds in one day after eating a certain food. It's not fat, but swelling and inflammation that can happen after you eat a food you're sensitive to.

One patient who was 25 years old and weighed 140 pounds was very sensitive to gluten. She had been on the FreeDiet® for a while and was doing great. Her abdominal pain, vomiting, fatigue, migraines, and skin issues had all cleared up. Then she had one small piece of chocolate cake not thinking it was such a big deal—and the next morning she was seven pounds heavier! This is not fat, but swelling and inflammation from eating a food she was sensitive to. Within three to four days, she dropped back down but didn't want to repeat that again!

One thing that can help when you're following the FreeDiet® is to only eat breakfast, lunch, and dinner. It's best to avoid snacking if you can so that you can give your blood sugar and insulin levels a chance to stay down for longer periods. This helps you burn fat. Also, avoid eating three hours before bedtime.

As far as exercise, high-intensity interval training is very effective for increasing your metabolism. See the FreeDiet® Fitness Chapter 8 for more information on this.

Another patient, a 55-year-old woman named Louise, came in with hypothyroidism, fatigue, brain fog, chronic pain, insomnia, digestive symptoms, and inability to lose weight. The only way she had been able to lose weight was under her doctor's recommendation of consuming only 500 calories per day and running seven to ten miles almost daily. Even then, the weight loss stopped, and she was only able to maintain her current weight. When she injured her back and had to stop running, she quickly gained 20 pounds and was feeling miserable.

After doing initial lab work and putting her on the FreeDiet®, she lost ten pounds in the first four weeks, and all her symptoms improved dramatically. No more counting calories—in fact, she could eat three times as much as before.

It's not about the calories or exercise. It's about eating foods that are right for you and avoiding those foods that are causing harm to your body. That's why the FreeDiet® is so effective with weight loss. You're avoiding foods that are most commonly responsible for inflammation, autoimmune diseases, gut issues, and other chronic health conditions.

CHAPTER 17

THE FREEDIET® FIX FOR HIGH FERRITIN

There is a blood test called ferritin, which can represent the amount of iron that's stored in your body. If you are low in iron, you can get a whole lot of symptoms like fatigue, brain fog, anxiety, depression, headaches...just a whole host of symptoms that can make you feel terrible. High iron levels can also cause very similar symptoms and are very toxic to your body.

I had a patient years ago whose husband had hemochromatosis, which is a hereditary iron storage disease. He had ignored it for years, and by the time he had been officially diagnosed, the doctors didn't know how to help him. He spent months in the hospital, and he ended up dying from this. He was only in his 30s. This can be a very serious condition. Over one million people in the United States have iron overload or hemochromatosis. It's very simple to diagnose and treat if you do the right tests.

It is very important, the next time you get lab testing, to ask your doctor to order ferritin levels and iron profile (iron, percent saturation, TIBC) to make sure that you are okay in this area.

Besides iron overload or hemochromatosis, elevated ferritin can also be due to chronic alcohol consumption, fatty liver, inflammation, liver disease, viral hepatitis, malignancy, infection, metabolic syndrome, or diabetes. Thorough lab testing which includes an iron profile, CBC, chem panel, GGT, lipids, and CRP (see Chapter 10 for examples of the comprehensive health panel) is required to determine what is causing the high ferritin. You can also check for genetic markers for hemochromatosis if indicated. Even if they are positive, as with this patient, you can still lower ferritin levels. Your diet and lifestyle can influence your genes.

If you do have iron overload, it can damage your organs and joints. It can cause diabetes, arthritis, heart palpitations, arrhythmia, liver damage, fatigue, and many other symptoms.

As I mentioned earlier, I had a 32-year-old patient who was thin but had high blood pressure. He had fatigue, lack of focus and concentration, anxiety, lightheadedness, and heart palpitations (PVCs). His heart rate would be 120–150 beats per minute with palpitations and flutters. He had been to cardiologists and other doctors and had numerous tests. He wore a heart monitor at home, but they could never figure out what was causing it, so they put him on medications.

I did an evaluation and lab testing, which includes ferritin levels and other iron markers. His ferritin was 583 ng/ml—optimal ferritin levels are between 60–90 ng/ml. After eight weeks on the FreeDiet®, Natural Medicine Formulas, and regular infrared sauna use, his ferritin decreased to 118, his hypertension resolved, and his symptoms cleared up.

Iron overload can cause heart symptoms, gallbladder disease, depression, infertility, low testosterone, and cancer. The main symptoms of too much iron are lack of energy, abdominal pain, brain fog, heart flutters, fast heart rate, and loss of sex drive. Just overall feeling miserable. It can also cause joint pain, and it can lead to liver damage, cirrhosis, hepatitis, liver cancer, enlarged spleen, hypothyroidism, and hormone imbalances. Even neuro-degenerative diseases like early dementia, Parkinson's, Alzheimer's, ringing in the ears, vertigo—all these can be caused by iron overload.

Another patient, a 64-year-old woman, had been feeling miserable for over 20 years. She had been to several different doctors, had gallbladder surgery, pancreatitis, and pericarditis (heart inflammation). She was in the hospital multiple times, literally almost died. Ringing in the ears, vertigo, fatigue, brain fog, and many other symptoms on top of that—she was feeling completely miserable.

My initial evaluation included ferritin and iron profile. She was surprised, especially being a nurse, that no other doctors had ordered these tests.

Her levels were 1,094 ng/ml, and 60–90 is optimal! It was very serious, and she had elevated liver enzymes showing liver damage, high uric acid (which can damage the joints), increased CRP inflammatory marker, and several other lab values that were abnormal.

Treatment Options

The standard medical treatment is to do therapeutic phlebotomy. The challenge with that is that with every pint you donate you can only drop about 30 points of ferritin. At a certain point, you can become anemic and must stop for a while. She was able to donate blood three times in the first month before she then became severely anemic and couldn't donate anymore. Those three times would have brought it down only 90 points to 1,004. She had to get it down to around 100.

The protocol I used was:

The FreeDiet® with modifications of avoiding high iron foods, like liver, and limiting the intake of red meat. It's very important to avoid cast iron cookware and grill grates.

Natural Medicine Formulas including:
- ActivMulti™ without Iron—multivitamin
- OmegaSorb 3X™—high absorption fish oil
- D3 5000 + K2
- Magnesium Malate (Magnesium Citrate if have constipation)
- ProbioSupreme™30—probiotics
- Multi Minerals (w/o iron)
- Liver Support—formula with milk thistle, selenium, NAC, alpha lipoic acid
- Metal Cleanse™—oral chelating formula
- Curcumin Protect™—high absorption curcumin supplement

The FreeDiet® 3-Minute Super Smoothie, which includes FreeDiet™ Protein or Paleo Protein, FreeGreens™ Organic Superfood Powder, Organic Psyllium Husk Powder, and coconut oil, for nourishment and cleansing.

Infrared sauna (low EMF) three times per week, which helps eliminate toxins and heavy metals, including iron. Preheat sauna to 120 degrees Fahrenheit and turn up to 135 once in. Stay in for up to 30 minutes per your tolerance.

I also ran other tests that indicated leaky gut, yeast overgrowth, and gluten sensitivity, so I put her on other supplements to help heal her gut. Between the FreeDiet®, the sauna, and Natural Medicine Formulas, the program was very detoxifying and very cleansing. She started to feel better.

In four weeks, I checked her blood again. Her ferritin had dropped from 1,094 to 92, a drop of over 1,000 points! It was absolutely amazing. Her elevated liver enzymes also dropped over 60 percent to almost normal, and her CRP inflammatory marker decreased by 54 percent to normal levels. Uric acid and triglycerides came down to normal, too. All these levels dramatically improved in only four weeks.

Not only were her ferritin levels fine but her symptoms cleared up and she was feeling great, the best she felt in years! It just goes to show: The body has an incredible ability to heal itself.

If you find out the underlying root causes and provide the right course of action, the proper diet, supplementation, and lifestyle changes, you can get better. The human body is so amazing that you can heal almost any chronic health condition. You can get better.

CHAPTER 18

THE FREEDIET® FIX FOR HIGH BLOOD PRESSURE

O ver the 33-plus years that I've been in practice, I've seen count-less patients with high blood pressure. One thing they all seem to have in common is that they are on blood pressure medication.

When I check their blood pressure, it's high even though they're on blood pressure medication/s. I ask them why—if they have hypertension and they're on medication for it—do they still have high blood pressure? This doesn't make any sense.

Once starting medication for hypertension, the body begins to adapt to it, and before you know it you're prescribed a second medication. Your body is continually adapting because you're not getting to the root cause of the hypertension. Instead, you're just covering it up with medication and trying to force the blood pressure down. I had one patient tell me how concerned she was because her husband was on five different blood pressure medications, and he still had high blood pressure—despite being a cardiologist!

Almost 50 percent of Americans have high blood pressure. Most cases are primary hypertension, of which they say there is no known cause. Prior to 2017, hypertension was classified as a blood pressure (BP) reading of 140/90 mm Hg or higher, but the new guideline classifies it as 130/80 mm Hg or higher.

If you're 130/80, that's stage one hypertension—despite being a cardiologist!, which means that millions more Americans now qualify to be put on medication for hypertension. The usual recommendations—

eating a healthy diet, maintaining a healthy weight, getting enough physical activity, not smoking, limited alcohol use—if those worked, then more than 100 million U.S. adults wouldn't have hypertension.

Instead of the usual recommendations, we're going to talk about a few solutions that can help address the underlying root causes. These are the most common I see.

Deficiencies:
- Vitamin B12
- Folate
- Magnesium
- Vitamin D

In addition to the Functional Five:
- ActivMulti™ without Iron—multivitamin
- OmegaSorb 3X™—fish oil
- D3 5000 + K2
- Magnesium Malate (Magnesium Citrate if have constipation)
- ProbioSupreme™30—probiotics

And depending on lab test findings:
- B12 Supreme™—sublingual methylcobalamin 5000 mcg
- MethylFolate B12 Plus—methylfolate with B12
- Zinc Glycinate
- C-Bioflavonoids 500—vitamin C with bioflavonoids
- Curcumin Protect™—high absorption curcumin supplement
- DHEA (if serum levels are below 100 and other factors)
- Cortisol Quencher™—if cortisol is too high
- Thyroid support (based on testing)

Toxins
- Iron overload
- High mercury levels

Recommended supplements:
- N-Acetyl Cysteine (NAC)
- Metal Cleanse™—oral chelating formula

Infrared sauna therapy 30 minutes two to three times per week at 120–135 degrees Fahrenheit.

Infections

Yeast and/or bacterial overgrowth in the intestines, parasites, Epstein-Barr virus and/or Cytomegalovirus can be a contributing cause.

Additional recommended supplements based on lab results:
- Yeast Defeat™
- Microb-Balance™
- ImmunoSilver™—silver solution
- Gut Immune Repair™ DF
- Monolaurin

Food Sensitivities

The FreeDiet®, which is free of the most common food allergens—those foods most responsible for inflammation, digestive issues, and other chronic health issues. Inflammation is a root cause of so many chronic diseases, including heart disease and hypertension.

As such, the FreeDiet® can help dramatically with supporting healthy blood pressure levels. I typically see on average a 30-point reduction in the first four weeks of Phase 1.

Although, I once saw a 54-year-old patient named Tony with a blood pressure reading of 182/108. He'd followed the guidelines to prevent hypertension—didn't smoke, drank alcohol only occasionally, wasn't overweight, exercised regularly, and had a pretty healthy diet—but it wasn't working.

He went to his primary doctor and a cardiologist, and they both told him he needed to go on high blood pressure medication and cholesterol medication. The cardiologist told him that it runs in the family, and there's no way to fix it with diet, so he'd spend the rest of his life on this medication. Tony didn't accept that. He was a healthy guy, and at the age of 54, he didn't want to be on medication for the rest of his life.

I did an evaluation and ran some lab tests, which revealed some nutritional deficiencies and food allergies, both of which can be common causes of inflammation and hypertension. Based on the patient's results, I put him on the FreeDiet®, along with Natural Medicine Formulas, to treat his specific deficiencies.

Four weeks into treatment, his readings were down to 111/71. He dropped 71 points in four weeks! He was down to normal blood pressure, and he also dropped seven pounds, even though he wasn't that overweight.

In addition, his cholesterol went down 34 points, and the other deficiencies that showed up in his lab work—like vitamin D, magnesium, and vitamin B12—improved. The best part was that he was off all his medication!

Besides the proper diet and supplements, structural health is important. Stress to the neck, upper back, and shoulders especially can cause a lot of tension, which can contribute to high blood pressure, difficulty sleeping, an inability to relax, and headaches.

I had another patient, a 68-year-old woman named Paula, who came in with neck pain into her shoulder and arm, back and joint pain, fatigue, brain fog, vertigo, insomnia, sinus congestion, digestive issues (including diarrhea and constipation), as well as high blood pressure.

She started on the FreeDiet® and Natural Medicine Formulas, including the Functional Five—ActivMulti™, Vitamin D 5000 with K2, Magnesium Malate, OmegaSorb 3X™ fish oil, ProbioSupreme™ 30—plus other supplements based on her specific lab results. She also received chiropractic care and manual therapy.

After four weeks of treatment, most of her pain and other symptoms cleared up. She was sleeping through the night, and her blood pressure dropped 66 points to normal levels. She also normalized her glucose, triglycerides, and inflammation markers while losing 12 pounds in the process.

Whether it's hypertension, fatigue, anxiety, digestive issues, or other chronic health issues you're having, it doesn't necessarily mean you have to be on medication to cover up the symptoms and not fix the problem. If you're the type of person who wants to get to the root cause, really understand what's going on, and find specific solutions to get better, know that it's possible.

Almost every health problem has a solution; it's just a matter of getting to the root cause. You can often find solutions and clear these things up. Remain hopeful. You can get better.

CHAPTER 19

THE FREEDIET® RECIPES

N ow the fun part begins—making art out of protein, vegetables, and healthy fats. On our recipe site, SpoonfulofHealth.com, my wife, Dawn Rofrano, has created many delicious recipes, with beautiful pictures and a story behind each one.

I summarized some of the FreeDiet™ phase 1 recipes here. Visit our website to select additional FreeDiet™ Phase 1 or Phase 2 recipes.

Breakfast

To reiterate from chapter 3, the best breakfast during FreeDiet® Phase 1 and Phase 2 is a protein smoothie. It's fast, easy, and a great way to start your day. I call it the FreeDiet® 3-Minute Super Smoothie.

It is a great source of protein, fruits and vegetables, healthy fats, and fiber, and it only takes three minutes to make.

The FreeDiet® 3-Minute Super Smoothie recipe

Ingredients:
- 12 oz. water
- ½ cup frozen organic cherries or blueberries
- 1 serving FreeDiet™ Protein or organic pea protein
- 1 scoop FreeGreens™ Organic Superfood Powder
- 1 Tbsp. ground flaxseeds
- 1 tsp. Organic Psyllium Husk Powder gradually increasing to 1 Tbsp. over 1–2 weeks
- 1 Tbsp. organic unrefined coconut oil

1. Blend the water and organic cherries or blueberries for 5 seconds.

2. Then add the protein, FreeGreens™ Organic Superfood Powder, ground flaxseeds, psyllium, and coconut oil, and blend for another 5 seconds.

3. See the video at nmcwellness.com/dr-toms-3-minute-super-smoothie-recipe for how to make it.

Note:

- If you add everything at once and blend, it can get too thick with the psyllium. The same goes if you over blend. Simply follow the instructions above for the best results.

- For a more filling meal as well as some crunch, you can add dehydrated coconut chips and/or soaked nuts at the end and blend for a few seconds.

- For nut milk instead of water, use a handful of soaked nuts (especially cashews) or coconut chunks and add to 12 oz. water initially. Blend well before adding the fruit and powders.

- At any time if the smoothie is too thick, add more water.

- The 3-Minute Super Smoothie is an important part of the FreeDiet® since it's a great source of protein, fruits and vegetables, healthy fats, and fiber. It's both very nourishing and very cleansing. If you're in an area where you don't have the ingredients available to you and are unable to make a smoothie, a less preferable option is to have leftovers from dinner or have soaked raw nuts and coconut with berries.

Lunch/Dinner

You don't have to be bored of the same old food day after
steak, fish with vegetables. Here are some amazing recipes that .
Dawn, put together that give you a lot of variety and scrumptious tas.

Soups

Healing Chicken Soup

Ingredients
- 1 whole chicken
- 4 stalks celery
- 1 whole head garlic
- 1 medium onion
- 2 strips or 2 Tbsp. of kelp

- 1 handful chives
- 1 bundle parsley
- 2 chunks ginger (2" x 2")
- Few dashes of oregano
- 2 tsp. pink Himalayan salt

Instructions
1. In a large pot filled halfway with water, add whole chicken and gently boil for 20 minutes.
2. Make sure chicken is covered with water. Add 2 tsp. of salt.
3. Wash and cut all vegetables.
4. Check chicken and skim off the white foam that is the chicken fat. Turn down to low heat after 20 minutes.
5. Add celery, onions, ginger, garlic, oregano, and cook for another 20 minutes.
6. At this point, you can lift the chicken out and separate meat to add back to the soup.
7. Add the chopped parsley, oregano, and kelp just before it is done.
8. Additional salt to taste if desired and enjoy the natural healing properties of this soup!

tes from Dawn

he secret to this soup being what I call "the world's most healing soup" is the ginger, kelp, whole head of garlic, and oregano. You can freeze any leftovers in small glass jars for when the need arises. Make sure to leave a few inches from the top to allow for expansion when freezing. Please use all organic ingredients in this soup when you can.

Creamy Butternut Soup

Ingredients

- 1 large butternut squash or 2 frozen 16 oz. bags
- 8 cups water
- 6 garlic cloves
- 1½ cups soaked cashews
- ½ cup hemp seeds
- 1 can coconut milk (full fat)
- 1 large onion
- 8-10 scallion stalks
- 1 tsp. ground cumin
- 1 tsp. turmeric
- 2½ tsp. pink Himalayan sea salt
- ½ tsp. ground cayenne (omit for FreeDiet® Phase 1)
- 2 tsp. ground curry (omit for FreeDiet® Phase 1)
- pepper to taste (omit for FreeDiet® Phase 1)

optional:
- 1 strip kelp

Instructions

1. If you bought a whole butternut squash, poke holes in it and bake/steam 30 minutes until soft enough to cut.
2. After it cools, cut into chunks and add to water with garlic, onions, scallions, spices, salt, and kelp.
3. If you used frozen squash, add those into the pot with the above.
4. Simmer for 20 minutes.
5. Add coconut milk and hemp seeds, turning off heat.
6. In small batches transfer mixture to a strong blender, like the Vitamix, and puree until creamy. Or better yet, use a handheld mixer in the pan.
7. Add everything back into the pot and stir, adding more salt, pepper, or spices to your taste.

Notes

If time is of the essence, you can use frozen butternut squash. Having to bake or steam the squash will add extra time to this recipe. Also, you can soak the cashews overnight or at least three hours to use in this soup. Soaking the cashews lends to the creamy texture of this soup. Please use organic ingredients when you can.

Thai Cauliflower Soup

Ingredients
- 4 cups filtered water
- 1 large or 2 small heads cauliflower
- 4 stalks celery
- 1 chopped white onion
- 1 bag frozen butternut squash (16–20 oz.)
- 1 15 oz. can coconut milk
- 5 cloves garlic
- 4-5 tsp. pink Himalayan sea salt
- 3 Tbsp. coconut oil
- 1 tsp. cumin
- 1 tsp. turmeric powder
- 1 tsp. chopped ginger root
- ¼ tsp. ground cardamom
- 1 tsp. curry*
- ¼ tsp. ground black pepper*
- optional dash cayenne* or red pepper*
- *omit for the FreeDiet® Phase 1

Instructions
1. In a large pot, boil water with chopped cauliflower, celery, garlic, onion, ginger, and turmeric roots, squash, and salt.
2. After a few minutes, the vegetables will soften a little. Turn heat down to low and let simmer.
3. Add turmeric powder, curry, cumin, coconut oil, and milk.
4. Reserve 1½ cups of vegetables and puree the rest of the soup. Combine both and serve.

Notes
Use organic ingredients when you can.

Entrées

Artichoke Encrusted Fish

Ingredients

- 3–6 pieces of fish
- 1 jar or bag of frozen artichoke hearts (6–9)
- juice of 1 lemon
- ½ cup of shredded coconut
- 1 Tbsp. coconut oil
- 1 tsp. of Himalayan pink sea salt
- 1 tsp. dill

Instructions

1. In a food processor, blend all the ingredients (except fish) until creamy.
2. Taste and add more salt if needed.
3. Spread a few Tbsp. of mixture equally on top of fish of your choice.
4. You can reserve ½ cup of mixture to also make a creamy sauce. *See notes.
5. Bake at 350 degrees Fahrenheit or 15–18 minutes or until fish is done.
6. Broil for 3–5 more minutes if you would like the top browned.

Notes

The artichoke mixture tastes great on white fish or salmon! You can make the crust as thick or thin as you like. I have also made a sauce in the blender to drizzle over the fish; *by reserving ½ cup of the mixture and add 2 Tbsp. olive oil, ¼ cup water, 2 Tbsp. of lemon juice. The leftover sauce we used as a dip or on salad. Frozen artichokes are first choice, followed by glass jars and then canned. Please buy wild-caught fish if possible.

Salmon Cakes

Ingredients

- 1½ lbs. salmon (about 4 pieces)
- 1 small red pepper or for FreeDiet® Phase 1, use 2 celery stalks
- ½ cup shredded unsweetened coconut
- 2 Tbsp. fresh or dried chives
- 1 tsp. pink Himalayan sea salt
- ¼ tsp. garlic powder
- ½ tsp. onion powder
- ¼ cup ground flax
- 1 lemon's juice

See recipe below for Creamy Cashew Sauce

Instructions

1. Put a large frying pan on medium heat with a few inches of water. Steam salmon until slightly underdone.
2. Let the salmon cool and peel any skin off.
3. Finely chop red pepper (or celery) and chives. Add to a big bowl, set aside.
4. Juice the lemon in a bowl and add ground flaxseeds, stir and let sit a few minutes until it gels.
5. In a food processor, add cooled skinless, boneless salmon, salt, onion and garlic powder. Pulse until it is fine texture.
6. In the large bowl with red pepper and chives, add salmon, coconut, flax/lemon, and mix well.
7. Oil a baking sheet or stoneware and form 8 cakes. Bake for 10 minutes.
8. To brown the cakes, broil for 5 minutes. Drizzle Creamy Cashew Sauce over cakes and enjoy!

Notes

For the FreeDiet® Phase 1, omit the red pepper and use 2 celery stalks chopped fine. Please use wild fish when you can and for a mild salmon, try Keta salmon. Be sure to pulse fish well so it is almost the consistency of tuna salad. This is key to the cakes holding their shape. To freeze, completely cool, wrap in wax paper, and tuck into a Ziploc bag.

Reheat in a pan with few tsps. water on low heat or thaw and pan fry for 5 minutes.

Creamy Cashew Sauce

Ingredients
- 1 cup of raw cashews with filtered water to fill jar
- ½ cup filtered water
- ¼ cup lemon juice
- ½ tsp. pink Himalayan sea salt
- ⅛ tsp. garlic powder
- 1 Tbsp. extra virgin olive oil
- 1 tsp. onion flakes or powder

Instructions
1. Fill a glass jar or bowl with filtered water that fills over the cashews. Soak nuts for at least 3 hours, and preferably overnight if you have the time. Drain and rinse cashews.
2. In a strong blender, add ½ cup filtered water, lemon juice, olive oil, spices, and soaked cashews.
3. Blend for a few minutes until consistency is creamy smooth.

Citrus Crusted Cod

Ingredients

- 4 pieces of cod
- juice of a lemon
- ¼ cup coconut flour
- ½ tsp. pink Himalayan sea salt
- 3 Tbsp. onion flakes
- 3 Tbsp. coconut or avocado oil
- extra oil for pan

Instructions

1. Soak fish in lemon juice, flipping it on each side.
2. In a large frying pan, heat 3 Tbsps. coconut or avocado oil on medium heat.
3. In a bowl, blend coconut flour, salt, and onion flakes.
4. Place a piece of fish in flour mixture and press mixture into each side.
5. When you see arcs on the side of the pan or the oil sizzles, place coated fish pieces in.
6. Let each piece cook and brown for a few minutes on each side.
7. Try not to peek, as moving the fish will make the coating fall off if it is not ready.
8. When fish seems firm and edges are nicely brown, flip each piece gently.

Notes

You can use any white fish, but this recipe works best with thinner fillets. The onion flakes are key to this recipe. If you cannot find Simply Organic brand onion flakes, you can use another brand if it is only onion flakes without other additives.

Another "citrus" twist on this fish is using the juice of an orange instead of lemon, but not for the FreeDiet® Phase 1.

Also, see recipe below or click link for Creamy Chive and Garlic Dressing to dip this fish in for that extra gourmet touch. It is not necessary to make dressing but super simple and, oh, so good!

Please use wild-caught fish and organic ingredients when you can.

Hazelnut Encrusted Flounder with Mango Mint Chutney

Ingredients
- 8 thin white fish fillets
- ½ cup hazelnuts or pecans
- ½ cup shredded coconut
- 4 Tbsp. coconut oil
- 1 tsp. sea salt
- ½ lime's juice

Mango Chutney (omit for FreeDiet® Phase 1)
- 1 ripe mango
- 1½ lime's juice
- ½ cup coconut cream
- handful of fresh mint
- sea salt dash
- pepper dash
- nutmeg dash

Instructions

1. In a food processor or strong blender, finely ground the nuts.
2. In a bowl, mix nut flour, shredded coconut, coconut oil, and sea salt. Set aside.
3. Lay fish in a large casserole dish so they are not overlapping and squeeze lime juice on top.
4. Cover fish with nut mixture and bake for 20–25 minutes in a 350-degree oven until it is golden brown.
5. While fish is cooking, cut mango into small pieces and chop mint finely.
6. Toss the lime juice, mango, mint, coconut milk, pepper, sea salt, and nutmeg in a bowl.
7. When encrusted fillets are done baking, spoon a few Tbsps. of chutney over fish while on a plate.

Notes

I like to use a mild fish so that I can taste the flavors of the encrusted topping. Purchase wild-caught seafood when possible. For a nut-free version, pumpkin seeds work nicely.

Basil and Artichoke Stuffed Chicken with Cashew Cheese

Ingredients

- 4 chicken breasts
- 2 cups artichokes (frozen)
- handful of basil
- 3 cloves garlic
- 1 tsp. pink Himalayan sea salt
- 3 Tbsp. olive oil
- Italian spices
- garlic powder

Optional creamy cashew cheese sauce:

- See recipe under Salmon Cakes earlier in this chapter.

Instructions

1. In a food processor or blender, pulse artichokes, basil, garlic, olive oil, and salt until blended.
2. Using sharp scissors or a knife, slice open the chicken breast ¾ through and place in a baking dish.
3. Season the top of chicken with spices, garlic, and salt. Stuff the chicken with about ¼ cup filling.
4. Bake the chicken at 350 degrees Fahrenheit for 35 minutes or until juices run clear.
5. If using the cashew cheese sauce, drizzle a few tablespoons over the top and serve.

Notes

Using frozen artichokes is preferred, as they do not have any unwanted added ingredients or preservatives as do the artichokes in a can or jar. Thawing out the artichokes isn't necessary, but rinsing them with water is helpful. Broiling the chicken for the last few minutes is an option to give it a nice golden color. Please use organic when you can.

Coconut Crusted Chicken with Sweet Lime Sauce

Ingredients

Chicken
- Chicken tenders, approximately 1.5 lbs.
- 2 eggs (substitute olive, avocado, or coconut oil for the FreeDiet® Phase 1)
- 1/2 cup shredded unsweetened coconut
- 1/2 tsp. pink Himalayan sea salt
- 1 Tbsp. onion flakes or 1/2 tsp. onion powder
- 1/4 tsp. paprika *omit for the FreeDiet® Phase 1

Sweet Lime Sauce:
- juice of 2 limes
- 3 Tbsp. shredded coconut
- 1/2 cup melted coconut oil
- 1/4 tsp. cumin
- 1/16 tsp. stevia (or few dashes to desired sweetness)

Instructions
1. Preheat oven to 350.
2. In a medium bowl, add shredded coconut, salt, paprika, and onion flakes.
3. In a separate small bowl, add eggs and beat them (unless you're substituting oil).
4. Take thin tenderloins and dip them in the egg (or oil), coating them well on both sides.
5. Dip each piece into the shredded coconut mixture and place in a baking dish.
6. Bake at 350 for 15–18 minutes until they are golden. Keep in mind, if they are thicker, then increase cooking time.

Sweet Lime Sauce:

In a blender, add all ingredients for sauce and mix until it is creamy.

Notes

You can store the unused sauce in the fridge. It will harden but will soften at room temperature, or you can heat it gently when ready to use.

I love that my sweet lime sauce is sugar-free and has a tangy bite to it! Keep in mind stevia is super strong, so a little goes a long way. Or you can use monk fruit instead. If you use whole chicken breasts, cutting them into strips, then pressing them flat between wax paper and a heavy frying pan will work great. Please use organic ingredients when you can.

Avocado Curry Chicken Salad

Ingredients for salad

- 1½ lbs. cooked chicken (about 3 breasts)
- 1 apple
- 3 celery stalks
- handful of basil or mint
- 1–2 tsp. curry powder
- ½ tsp. pink Himalayan sea salt
- dash cumin

Ingredients for Dressing:

- ½ cup soaked cashews
- 1 small or ½ large avocado
- juice of 2 lemons
- ½ cup olive oil or avocado oil
- 2 tsp. pink Himalayan sea salt
- 1 tsp. onion powder

Instructions

1. Soak cashews at least 3 hours. Overnight is best for the dressing.
2. Chop and shred cooked and cooled chicken and place in a bowl.
3. Chop celery and apple and add to the shredded chicken.
4. Chop mint or basil and add to bowl.
5. In a strong blender, like the Vitamix, add all dressing ingredients and mix.
6. Add about ½ cup dressing to chicken salad and blend. Add more if you desire.
7. Mix in the curry (add 1 tsp. at a time and taste), cumin, and salt to taste.

Notes

I have made the dressing without the avocado and just added more soaked cashews (a small handful). If you find the dressing is too thick, adjust it by adding some filtered water. If texture is too thin, add more cashews. This dressing is so versatile and can be used on salad, fish, or vegetables. It will stay fresh in the fridge up to 5 days. I love using leftover chicken or cooking chicken the night before and making the chicken salad the next day. If you love curry, go for the 2 tsp. cumin, and using the mint (versus the basil) balances the spicy flavor. Please use organic when you can.

Easy Meatloaf

Ingredients:
- 1 1/2 lbs. grass-fed beef
- 1 cup shredded zucchini (1 small zucchini)
- 1 Tbsp. Italian spices
- 1 tsp. sea salt plus a dash or two
- 1/4 tsp. garlic powder

Instructions
1. Preheat oven to 350 degrees.
2. Sprinkle a few dashes of sea salt over shredded zucchini.
3. Blend all the ingredients together.
4. Press the meat into loaf pan and spread pesto sauce on top.
5. Bake for 45 minutes or until done and let cool after draining the juices.

Tips:
For FreeDiet® Phase 2, you can use shredded white or sweet potato with salt and drizzle with olive oil. When potato bakes on top, it is crispy good! Careful not to overcook grass-fed beef, as it tends to be lean and cooks faster.

Paleo Meatballs

Ingredients

- 1½ lbs. grass-fed beef
- 1 small-medium zucchini
- 1 Tbsp. Italian spices
- 1 tsp. Himalayan/sea salt
- 1 Tbsp. onion flakes
- ½ tsp. garlic powder

Instructions

1. Preheat your oven to 350 degrees.
2. In a big bowl, add meat, spices, and salt.
3. Wash zucchini and, using the smallest shredding side of your grater (with skin on), shred zucchini.
4. Add to the meat and blend all ingredients.
5. Using about 2 rounded Tbsps., roll meat into balls in the palm of your hand, or use an ice cream scoop.
6. You can make them smaller (and have more for appetizers), but you will need to adjust the time.
7. Be careful not to overcook the grass-fed beef.

Notes

These meatballs are moist because of the zucchini. When rolling the meatballs in your hands, they will be soft but will firm up after baking them. Please use organic ingredients when you can.

Steak Fajitas

Ingredients

- 1½ lbs. beef sirloin flap
- 8 grain-free wraps
- 1 Tbsp. coconut oil
- 2 small onions
- 3 red bell peppers or for

the FreeDiet® Phase 1, use julienned zucchini
- ½ tsp. pink Himalayan sea salt
- handful of chives

Guacamole Marinade:

- 2 limes
- 6 garlic cloves
- 1 tsp. ground cumin
- ½ tsp. pink Himalayan sea salt

Instructions

1. In a large bowl, squeeze two limes. Add cumin and salt to the lime juice.
2. Chop garlic cloves into fine pieces and cut sirloin flap into long, thin chunks.
3. Put meat and garlic in the large glass bowl with lime juice and spices.
4. Let this marinate for as long as you can.
5. Chop the onions, peppers, and sauté them with coconut oil.
6. Heat up the wraps and spread guacamole and add few strips of steak and vegetables.
7. Careful not to overfill your wrap. Fold bottom up first and then sides.

Notes

If you are on the FreeDiet® Phase 1, you can use coconut wraps (turmeric flavor or plain) that work well. Although the Siete brand that I love has very few ingredients, the apple cider vinegar is a food to avoid while on the FreeDiet® Phase 1. You can omit the red peppers and substitute julienned zucchini or another FreeDiet® approved vegetable.

Please use organic ingredients and grass-fed beef when possible.

Cauliflower Fried Rice

Ingredients

- 10–12 oz. frozen bag riced cauliflower or 1 head cauliflower riced
- 4 large scallion shoots
- ½ tsp. pink Himalayan sea salt
- 3 tsp. dried onion flakes
- 3 Tbsp. avocado oil

Instructions

1. Chop green onion shoots.
2. In a large bowl, add riced cauliflower, scallions, and spices.
3. In a large frying pan, add oil and heat to low-medium.
4. When pan sizzles when a drop of water hits the pan, add cauliflower rice to pan.
5. Cover and cook for 5–8 minutes until golden brown.
6. With a large spatula, flip rice so other side can brown slightly and cook 5–8 minutes.
7. Serve warm or store in fridge to reheat.

Notes

Most markets carry frozen riced cauliflower, but you can make your own by chopping it into chunks and pulsing it in a food processor. I often make a double batch for leftovers. Also, in FreeDiet® Phase 2, if you are okay with eggs, then adding one to this recipe gives it that authentic fried rice flair! Just crack it in the middle of your pan with the riced cauliflower and stir. As an option, you can use coconut oil for a sweeter flavor. For onion flakes, I prefer Simply Organic brand.

Please use organic ingredients when you can.

Cauliflower Cakes

Ingredients

- 2 cup finely ground/riced cauliflower
- ¼ cup hemp seeds
- ½ cup ground flax
- ½ cup water

- 2 Tbsp. melted coconut oil
- 1 Tbsp. onion flakes
- 1 tsp. ground oregano
- 1 tsp. ground basil
- 1 tsp. pink Himalayan sea salt

Instructions

1. In a bowl, add the water, oil, and flax. Stir until it forms into a gel. Set aside.
2. In a food processor or blender, add the remaining ingredients.
3. Add the flaxseed mixture into the above ingredients and mix until blended.
4. Using an ice cream scoop or 2 Tbsps. mixture in hands to form a ball.
5. Place them on a baking sheet an inch apart and flatten with palm of hand.
6. Bake 25 minutes in a 350-degree oven or until the edges are golden.
7. This version will not brown as much as the one with cheese.
8. Please let them cool before serving so they can set.

Notes

I love the convenience of buying the frozen riced cauliflower, but I have also finely ground up a small head of cauliflower in my food processor. You can freeze any leftover riced cauliflower. I don't suggest buying the pre-cut florets in a bag unless it is frozen. They lose their freshness and nutrients after cut unless frozen right away. Texture will be different, but it bakes fine. Make sure to flatten with your palm so they bake well. Please use organic ingredients when you can.

Zucchini Cakes

Ingredients

- 1 zucchini
- 1 cup "soaked" raw pumpkin seeds *
- 1/2 cup finely shredded coconut
- 2 Tbsp. ground flaxseeds
- 2 Tbsp. coconut oil
- 3 stems of chives
- 10 leaves of Italian parsley
- 1/4 tsp. sea salt to taste
- 3 tsp. water

Instructions

1. Using a Vitamix or food processor, grind pumpkin seeds (doesn't have to be fine).
2. Shred zucchini and add water. Add pumpkin seeds into the bowl.
3. Wash and chop chives and Italian parsley.
4. Blend all the other ingredients in the bowl and add shredded zucchini.
5. Form about 3 Tbsp. into 6–7 small patties and bake at 350 for 25 minutes or until golden on edges.

Notes:

Let the ingredients sit for a few minutes after you blend them. This will give time for the flaxseeds to absorb and gel everything together. Take note: If you cook in a convection oven versus regular bake, this cooks the cakes differently. When using regular bake, adding a Tbsp. of olive oil will help keep them moist.

*Soaking pumpkin seeds makes all the difference (see snacks in this chapter for how).

I think doubling the batch makes sense so you can freeze these cakes for easy reheating.

Zucchini Noodles with Creamy Cashew Sauce

Ingredients

- 1 cup of raw cashews
- filtered water to fill jar
- ½ cup filtered water
- ¼ cup lemon juice
- ½ tsp. pink Himalayan sea salt
- ⅛ tsp. garlic powder
- 1 Tbsp. extra virgin olive oil
- 1 tsp. onion flakes or powder
- 2 large zucchinis
- 2 Tbsp. coconut oil
- 1 Tbsp. Italian spices
- ¼ tsp. pink Himalayan sea salt

Instructions

1. Fill a glass jar or bowl with filtered water that fills over the cashews. Soak nuts preferably overnight if you have the time. Drain and rinse cashews.
2. In a strong blender, add ½ cup filtered water, lemon juice, olive oil, salt, garlic, onion flakes/powder, and soaked cashews.
3. Blend for a few minutes until consistency is creamy smooth.
4. Taste and add any extra sea salt as desired. Will keep up to a week refrigerated.
5. To make the zucchini noodles, you will need a spiralizer (see resource section), or you can chop them however you like.
6. In a large frying pan, add coconut oil and sauté noodles on medium heat with spices.
7. After a few minutes, check to see if they are al dente and add ¼ cup of cashew sauce.
8. Stir and take off the heat immediately.

Notes

If time is of the essence, you can soak the cashews for 1½ hours, but I find the longer they soak the creamier the sauce. I love using this sauce on my salads—in fact, you may notice it resembles many of my salad dressing recipes. You can also have the kids dip some cut-up vegetables in it! Please use organic when you can.

Snacks

For most people, I recommend only three meals per day. The FreeDiet®
3-Minute Super Smoothie for breakfast, and then lunch and dinner. If
you need to have a midmorning and/or a midafternoon snack, then I
recommend:

Soaked Nuts

How to Soak Nuts
Place raw nuts into a glass jar or bowl.
Cover with filtered water, by at least ½ inch over the top of nuts (because
they expand).
Add 1 Tbsp. of salt per quart of water as an option.
Leave on the counter for 12–24 hours.

You can then change water and place it in the refrigerator, where you can
keep nuts for up to five days if you change the water daily.
For nut milk and recipes, you can use the soaked nuts without dehydrating
or roasting.

To dry the nuts:
You can sprinkle some Himalayan or sea salt over the nuts beforehand.
For pecans, cinnamon with monk fruit or stevia powder tastes great.
If you have a dehydrator, spread them out on the trays and dehydrate at
120 degrees Fahrenheit for 24 to 48 hours, until crisp.
Or place in oven at the typical lowest setting, which is 175–200 degrees
Fahrenheit. Depending on the temperature you choose and the type of
nut, bake/roast for 4–10 hours or until crisp. You can use a higher tem-
perature if you want them done faster.

Nut Milk

Soaked nuts are great for making nut milk. This is so much healthier and less expensive than buying nut milk. Simply take a handful of soaked nuts and put it in 8 to 12 ounces of water in the Vitamix or strong blender and turn on high for about 10 seconds. There you have it, fresh nut milk in seconds. You can also add some berries, monk fruit, or stevia for sweetness, or vanilla extract.

For the FreeDiet® 3-Minute Super Smoothie, you can also add some soaked nuts to the water in the beginning. This way, you're using nut milk instead of water.

View this quick video to learn more about soaking nuts at nmwellness.com/how-and-why-to-soak-nuts/.

The FreeDiet® 3-Minute Super Smoothie

You can have a 2nd complete smoothie or a variation of, like just the protein in water.

FreeGreens™ Organic Superfood Powder

Simply mix in water for a quick pick me-up. Some call it their green coffee.

(Un) Creamy Artichoke Dip

Ingredients
- 1 bag frozen artichokes
- 1 cup soaked cashews
- 2 Tbsp. lemon juice
- 2 Tbsp. olive oil
- handful parsley or basil
- handful of fresh chives or 2 Tbsp. dried chives
- 1 Tbsp. dried onion flakes
- 1 tsp. Himalayan salt
- 1/8 tsp. of garlic powder
- Celery, cucumber or jicama for dipping
- pepper to taste (omit for FreeDiet® Phase 1)

Instructions
1. Put all ingredients, except the fresh herbs, in blender like Vitamix or a food processor.
2. Puree until creamy and add fresh herbs, then pulse, taste, and add extra salt or pepper.
3. Cut some celery, cucumber, and or jicama and dip away!

Notes
Frozen artichoke hearts are preferable, as it is difficult to find canned artichokes without all the preservatives and salt. However, I did find Whole Foods 365 brand soaked in water. You will only need 8–9 whole artichokes for this recipe. I have played with adding rosemary or other herbs, and it tastes great.

Kale Chips with Ranch–O–Yum Dressing

Ingredients
- 2 small bunches green and purple kale
- 1/4 cup coconut oil
- 1/8 tsp. sea salt
- few dashes black pepper (omit for FreeDiet® Phase 1)
- Ranch-O-Yum Dressing (see salad dressing section for recipe)

Instructions
1. Preheat oven to 300 degrees.
2. Rinse kale and break away from stem into mouth-size pieces.
3. Dry well and place on a cookie sheet.
4. Mix salt and pepper into oil and toss kale in oil, rubbing all the leaves well.
5. Bake for 15 minutes in oven, tossing kale at least once so they do not burn.

Salad Dressings

As an option to olive oil with lemon or salt on your salad, here are some delicious dressing recipes from my wife, Dawn. The Zesty Lemon Dressing is especially delicious. Our daughter, at age eight years old, loved it so much that she would ask to have salad for a snack. Can you imagine your kid asking you to make a salad?

If you're getting tired of just chicken with vegetables or salmon with vegetables, you can use this dressing to make the plainest meal taste amazing. You can also add variety by using the dressing with your leftovers. For instance, if you have salmon leftovers the next day for lunch, you can make salmon salad with dressing. Instead of complaining about getting leftovers for lunch, you have a brand-new, delicious meal.

Zesty Lemon Dressing

Ingredients
- 1 cup olive oil
- 1 cup soaked cashews
- 3 lemons juiced (about 2/3 cup)
- 1½ tsp. pink Himalayan sea salt
- ½ tsp. onion powder
- few extra dashes

optional:
- 3 steamed garlic cloves

Instructions
1. Soak cashews at least 3 hours but overnight is best.
2. Rinse nuts well before you add them to make dressing.
3. Juice lemons; you should have about 2/3 cup. You can use limes if you are sensitive to lemons.
4. Add soaked nuts, lemon juice, oil, and spices to a strong blender until all is creamy.
5. Serve over salad, fish, or chicken, or dip raw vegetables into the dressing.

Notes
If you are adding the garlic, steam it gently in a saucepan. I prefer cooked garlic, as adding it raw is overpowering. This dressing is the base of many of my dressings, so have fun and add a little spice or other herbs, like chives! If you find your dressing is too thick, add a tad more water. If it is too thin, add a few extra nuts. Honestly, you can't go wrong here. I have tried this recipe with large lemons—it was tart, so I added more water. You can use avocado oil if you do not like the flavor of olive oil, or you can use a blend of them to equal a cup of oil. Please use organic when you can and cold-pressed extra virgin oils. This dressing will stay fresh for up to a week in the refrigerator if you don't eat it all at first!

Creamy Chive and Garlic Dressing

Ingredients

- 1 cup avocado or olive oil
- ¼ cup soaked cashews
- handful of baby chives
- 1 tsp. Himalayan pink sea salt
- 2 lemons juice
- 1 tsp. onion flakes
- ¼ tsp. garlic powder or
- 2 steamed garlic cloves

Instructions

1. In ¼ cup water, steam the garlic until it is soft.
2. In a strong blender, cream the oil, lemon juice, and soaked cashews.
3. Add all the other ingredients and blend until it is creamy.
4. Taste and add extra salt if needed to your liking.

Notes

I steam the garlic because it creates a milder flavor and makes it easier to digest. If you would like a thinner dressing, you can add a few Tbsps. of the water you steamed the garlic in. This dressing is also a great dip for baked chips or sliced vegetables. Drizzle it on fish or in your chicken salad instead of mayonnaise. The dressing will stay fresh up to a week in the refrigerator. Please use organic where you can.

Ranch-O-Yum Dressing

Ingredients

- ½ cup soaked cashews or macadamias
- ½ cup olive oil
- ½ cup cashew or coconut milk
- Juice of 1 lemon
- 2 Tbsp. coconut manna
- ½ tsp. sea salt
- ½ tsp. dill
- ⅛ tsp. garlic powder
- *few dash ground pepper
- *dash of paprika

*omit for FreeDiet® Phase 1

Instructions

1. In Vitamix or strong blender, add nuts, lemon juice, oil, and all spices and herbs.
2. Puree all ingredients until creamy.
3. Add extra salt to taste.

Notes

You can also use soaked walnuts as an option, and it will taste just as good! I have also used cashews that were not soaked, and it worked. But something about soaking the nuts helped with flavor and creaminess. It also helps our bodies to better digest the nuts when we soak them.

Pesto Sauce

Ingredients

- 1 cup raw pine nuts, soaked
- 2 lemon's juice
- 3/4 cup olive oil
- 4 full sprigs fresh basil
- 1 Tbsp. Italian spice
- 1 1/2 tsp. pink Himalayan or sea salt
- 1/4 tsp. onion powder

Instructions

1. If time permits, soak pine nuts for 8-plus hours. If time is of the essence, soak for at least a few hours.
2. In a strong blender, like the Vitamix, add nuts (soaked and rinsed), lemon juice, oil, spices, and fresh basil.
3. Blend until pesto is creamy smooth.
4. Pesto will stay fresh up to 5 days in the refrigerator. Use on fish, chicken, or salad!

Notes

If you prefer, you can also use soaked cashews or walnuts instead of pine nuts. If you have a nut allergy, you can substitute the pine nuts with pumpkin seeds. Follow the directions, but it is important to soak the seeds for this recipe. Lime juice is a great substitution if lemon is not an option. Please use organic when you can.

Desserts

Acai Gelatin Cups

Ingredients
- 3 raspberry tea bags
- 1 frozen pack acai fruit
- 4 cups filtered water
- 2 Tbsp. or packets gelatin powder
- 1 1/2 cups chopped fruit: cherries or blueberries (can also use strawberries in FreeDiet® Phase 2)
- 1/4 tsp. stevia or monk fruit

Instructions
1. Thaw out the acai pack of fruit by soaking in cold water for about 10 minutes.
2. Boil 2 1/2 cups of water and brew tea.
3. Put the other 1 1/2 cups room temperature water in a bowl.
4. Sprinkle gelatin over room temperature water and let it sit to bloom for a few minutes.
5. Sweeten the brewed tea with stevia or monk fruit and pour it over the bloomed gelatin.
6. Stir for a minute to allow the gelatin to activate with the hot tea.
7. Add chopped fruit, stir, and pour 1/2 cup servings into jars for easy on-the-go.
8. Refrigerate for a few hours until firm.

Notes
For approved fruit, use cherries or blueberries. I have used frozen and slightly thawed them without any repercussions with gelatin firming. Please chop the cherries. You may notice the acai fruit settles to the bottom but does not compromise taste or texture. Please use organic ingredients when you can.

Chai Cheesecake Bars

Filling:

- 2 1/2 cups soaked cashews
- 3/4 cup filtered water
- 2 scoops vanilla Paleo protein powder
- 2 Tbsp. coconut oil melted
- 1 Tbsp. gelatin or 1 packet
- 2 tsp. vanilla extract
- 2 tsp. stevia or monk fruit plus few dashes more to taste
- 1 1/2 Tbsp. ground cinnamon

Crust:

- 2 cups raw pecans (soaked)
- 1/4 tsp. pink Himalayan sea salt
- 1 tsp. maple extract
- 2 Tbsp. coconut oil
- 1/4 cup ground flaxseed
- 3 Tbsp. water
- Dash of stevia or monk fruit

Instructions

1. To make crust, preheat oven 350 degrees. Rinse off the pecans. Set aside in a bowl. In a cup, mix oil, maple extract, and toss over the pecans.
2. Toss pecans with 1/4 tsp. salt and bake nuts for 25 minutes.
3. To make filling, in a strong blender, cream the soaked cashews with all the ingredients. Set aside.
4. After pecans are baked, in a food processor or strong blender, pulse the nuts into a rough flour.
5. Add ground flaxseeds and dash salt. Pulse.
6. In a cup, mix water with few dashes of stevia or monk fruit powder and add to crust mixture, pulse until blended.
7. In an 11 x 9 (or so) glass dish, press the nut crust firmly into the dish. Crust should be packed tightly.
8. Chill for up to an hour in the freezer and then refrigerate. These bars can be cut and frozen, too.

Drinks

Natural Infused Water Recipes:

- Filtered water
- Handful of fresh basil
- 5 slices or more of cucumber
- Filtered water
- 1 lime
- few sprigs rosemary
- Filtered water
- raw ginger root, size of thumb
- 1 kiwi

- Filtered water
- 2 celery ribs (sticks)
- half pomegranate*
- Filtered water
- handful of fresh parsley
- few strawberries*
- 1 blood orange*
- juice of a boiled beet*

*omit for the FreeDiet® Phase 1

Instructions:

1. Wash all fruits, herbs, and vegetables. If you are using organic, leaving the skin on is fine.
2. Muddle the herbs to release the natural flavors gently.
3. Slice fruits and vegetables. Squeeze juice of lime, lemon, and orange into water.

Tips:

You can refill the infusions several times before discarding fruits, vegetables, and herbs. They will last in the refrigerator for a few days. Please use organic, especially when it comes to the Dirty Dozen (12 fruits/vegetables with the highest pesticide content per EWG.org).

I love slicing celery sticks and letting them soak in my glass water bottle to go!

Mixed Berry Juice

Ingredients
- 4½ cups water
- ½ cup fresh/frozen blueberries
- ½ cup fresh/frozen cherries
- 4 sprigs mint
- dash stevia leaf or monk fruit powder

Instructions
1. Add all washed ingredients to blender except stevia/monk fruit.
2. Blend for about 30 seconds and taste.
3. Add dash stevia or monk fruit powder to taste and blend for a few seconds.
4. With a fine strainer, separate seeds, if any, from berry juice.
5. Pour over ice, garnish with mint, and enjoy!

Notes
For the FreeDiet® Phase 1 and 2, we are keeping fruit sugar to a minimum, so a total of one serving/cup of fruit per day.
FreeDiet® Phase 2, you can use raspberries, strawberries, or blackberries. Using either the frozen berries will help juice to be chilled. Use stevia leaf powder from the whole leaf, as it is less refined.
Use organic ingredients and filtered water.

Cranberry Slushy

Ingredients
- 1/4 cup cranberries
- 1/2 cup cherries (frozen)
- 1 celery stalk
- 1/2 cup ice (4 cubes)
- 1 cup cold water
- handful parsley or mint
- optional: ginger, apple

Instructions
1. Add cranberries, cherries, celery, ice, water, and blend until creamy.
2. Add parsley or mint, blend 1 minute until a smooth slushy.
3. Drink up and feel SUPER!
4. *Remember for the FreeDiet® Phase 1 and 2, we are keeping fruit sugar to a minimum, so a total of one serving/cup of fruit per day.

CHAPTER 20

THE FREEDIET® FAST START—YOUR TIME TO BE FREE

I've covered lots of information, so I'm going to wrap this up for you so you can get off to a fast start.

1. Speak to members of your household and let them know what you're doing. Tell them why you are doing the FreeDiet® and what your goals are. Ask for their support in helping you stick with the program or even following it with you. Find out what their goals are.

   I had a 25-year-old patient who came to me with digestive and skin issues. At her first month follow-up, not only was she thrilled at how much better she was on the FreeDiet®, she said her mom lost 10 pounds and her dad lost 15 pounds in the process. They decided to support her by following it at the same time, and it paid off!

2. Clean out of your refrigerator and pantry of all foods on the avoid list. Either put them in a separate section if you have other household members that are eating them, give them away, or discard them. No sense in keeping forbidden foods in front of you that you will be tempted to eat.

3. Decide what meals you are going to have and circle the foods on the shopping list you will be eating for the next week—or less if you like to go to the store more often.

   Go shopping with the list and select your foods. Make sure to get frozen blueberries or cherries, unrefined coconut oil, and ground flaxseeds for your smoothie.

4. Prepare your meals for the day. You only need to make one meal— dinner with enough for leftovers the next day. To save time and make things easier, you can use an Instant Pot or Steam Convection Oven.

Here is a recap:

Breakfast—The FreeDiet® 3-Minute Super Smoothie

You will need:

- 12 oz. filtered water
- ½ cup frozen organic cherries or blueberries
- 1 serving FreeDiet™ Protein, Paleo protein, or organic pea protein
- 1 scoop FreeGreens™ Organic Superfood Powder
- 1 Tbsp. ground flaxseeds
- 1 tsp. Organic Psyllium Husk Powder gradually increasing to 1 Tbsp. over 1–2 weeks
- 1 Tbsp. organic unrefined coconut oil
- 1 blender to mix ingredients

Blend the water and organic cherries or blueberries for 5 seconds. Then add the protein, FreeGreens™, ground flaxseeds, psyllium, and coconut oil, and blend for another 5 seconds.

Lunch and Dinner

One of the following proteins: fish, chicken, turkey, beef, lamb (approx. 4 ounces) with plenty of vegetables and/or salad with extra virgin olive oil and lemon.

Best choices: wild fish, grass-fed beef, organic poultry

Midmorning or afternoon snacks (only if needed):

FreeGreens™ Organic Superfood Powder

The FreeDiet® 3-Minute Super Smoothie

Raw walnuts, cashews, pecans, hazelnuts, macadamia nuts, or Brazil nuts (soaked and dehydrated/roasted)

Raw vegetables with dressings/dips in Chapter 19.

Avoid all gluten, grains, sugar, yeast, dairy, eggs, soy, legumes, nightshades, and processed foods. This includes alcoholic beverages, vinegar, coffee, juices, soda, and sports drinks.

See the FreeDiet® Phase 1 food chart for a detailed list of the allowed and avoid foods.

Use sea salt or Himalayan salt, typically ½–1 tsp. daily.

5. Drink plenty of filtered water throughout the day, especially between meals. You can squeeze fresh lemon or lime in water if desired. A general recommendation is to drink at least half of your body weight in ounces. For example, a 140-pound person would drink 70 ounces (2 liters) of water. Drink more if engaging in outdoor activities or exercise that causes you to perspire.

6. Take the Functional Five supplements:

ActivMulti™ w/o iron—multivitamin

OmegaSorb3X™—fish oil capsules

D3 5000 + K2—most need 5000 IU/day of vitamin D

Magnesium Malate (or Citrate if you have constipation)

ProbioSupreme™ 30—probiotic

To save time, get a 7-day (3-4 times per day) pillbox, so you can enter all your supplements for the week. See naturalmedicineformulas.com for this and more information on supplements.

7. Walk each day for 15–30 minutes outside for stress relief and to clear

your mind.

8. Go to bed by 10 PM (11 PM the latest) and get up at 6 or 7 AM each day.
   Avoid electronics and screen time (phone, tablet, computer, TV) one hour before bed to help you sleep better.

9. Stick with this. It can be challenging for the first few days—establishing new routines and habits. You may experience withdrawal symptoms and be a bit irritable. Know that it will get better. By the end of the first week, most people start to notice more energy, less pain, clearer thinking, gut improving, etc.

10. Check in along the way. After the first 28 days, take the Health Assessment again and see how you score. See how many of your goals you have made progress toward. By focusing on the improvements, it encourages you to keep going.

One of the most rewarding experiences in my life is when I see the amazing lab result improvements in such a short time, and patients tell me how much better they are doing in so many different areas from being on the FreeDiet®.

They tell me:
"It's life-changing. I feel the best I have in years. I easily lost that stubborn weight and look better than I have in such a long time. I have more energy. My digestion has cleared up. My skin is better. I can think clearly now. I'm free of pain. My thyroid is better. My family and friends have noticed such a difference."

That's what I want for you. A life-changing experience. You can do this. You can get better. You can enjoy vibrant health and feel the best you have in years!

ACKNOWLEDGMENTS

I am thankful for:

My wife, Dawn, who has been at my side for the past 27 years. Thank you for creating the recipes for this book and on our website. You are a beautiful person, an amazing cook and creative, and I love you deeply.

My daughter, Adriana, who has inspired me to raise my level of contribution to this world. Plus, I've had so much fun with you doing our healthy cooking shows!

My mother, Jeanne Lochner, R.N., for guiding me in the direction of natural health and intuitively knowing which doors for me to go through.

My father, Douglas Rofrano, M.D., for sparking my early interest in health care and showing me what it's like to care for your patients.

Kayla, our patient care coordinator, for your loyalty and keeping things running smoothly at the Natural Medicine Clinic so that we can help so many transform their lives.

Peter Osborne for being a great coach and mentor.

The thousands of patients that I have been able to help and learn from over the past 33-plus years. I appreciate your trust and look forward to continuing to help you on your journey to achieve vibrant health!

APPENDIX

I often get asked how the FreeDiet® compares to other diets. So, I created this chart comparing some of the most popular diets, including the Paleo diet, Autoimmune Paleo, Candida diet, Bulletproof, Body Ecology, elimination diet, keto diet, FODMAP, and Whole30.

The Yes column contains foods allowed on that diet but not on the FreeDiet®.

The No column contains foods that are not allowed on that diet but are on the FreeDiet®.

The FreeDiet® Comparison Chart

Paleo		AIP		Candida diet	
Yes	No	Yes	No	Yes	No
Beer and Wine Spirits Diet soda Coffee	Salt	Kombucha Coconut yogurt and kefir Water kefir	Nuts Seeds Stevia Xylitol	Kombucha Yogurt Kefir Sauerkraut Kimchi	All fruit except lemon and lime
All the meat and fish and shellfish you can eat Eggs		Fermented vegetables Fermented fruit	Herbs from seeds	Almonds	Green tea Cashews
Mushrooms Peppers Eggplant Sweet potatoes Yams		All vegetables except night-shades		Spinach Tomatoes Eggplant Pickles Olives	
All the fruits you can eat		Vinegar: App cider, coconut, red wine, balsamic		Buckwheat Millet Oat bran Quinoa Teff	
Fruit w/ each meal Dried Fruits		1 tsp. honey and maple syrup		Black pepper Paprika	
Pistachios		Arrowroot starch		Apple cider vinegar Coconut aminos	
Vinegar					

Bulletproof		Body Ecology		Elimination Diet	
Yes	No	Yes	No	Yes	No
Coffee	Pea protein	Eggs	All fruit except lemon, lime, black currants, and cranberry	Mushrooms Sweet potato Yams Spinach Rhubarb Carrots Beets All vegetables except nightshades	Meat Poultry Fish
Eggs Tilapia Shellfish Pork Butter Cocoa Raw milk Cream Butter Raw yogurt Whey	Brazil nuts Pine nuts Flaxseed	Millet Amaranth Quinoa Buckwheat		Bananas Figs Grapes Melons Pineapple All fruit except citrus	Lemon Lime
White rice Cassava Plantain Sweet potatoes Yams		Raw beets, parsnips Sweet potatoes and Yams		Rice Buckwheat	Nuts Seeds
Carrots Spinach Tomatoes Olives		Red-skin potatoes		Black pepper	
Blackberries Raspberries Pineapple Strawberries Grapefruit Melons Citrus		Nuts and seeds except pumpkin seeds		Apple cider vinegar Coconut vinegar Rice milk	
Pistachios					
Apple cider vinegar Mustard Glucose Raw honey Chocolate					
Chocolate					

Whole30		Keto Diet		FODMAP	
Yes	No	Yes	No	Yes	No
Coffee Fruit juice Apple cider Kombucha Cacao	Stevia Xylitol Pea protein	Low-carb Kombucha and Alcohol Almond milk Soymilk Coffee Tea, black	Apples Papaya Peach- es Pears Plums Ca- shews	1 bottle beer 1 glass of wine 1 drink alcohol Diet sodas Fruit juice (mod- erate amt.)	Anise/ fennel Artichoke Avocado Asparagus Beets Broccoli Brussels sprouts Cabbage Cauliflower Celery Garlic Leeks Onions
Bananas Dates Figs Grapefruit Grapes Mango Melon Oranges Pineapple Plantains Strawberries Tangerines Watermelon		Beef jerky Pork Pork rinds Bacon Cold cuts Hot dogs Sausage Shellfish Tuna Canned meats Canned fish Eggs		Coffee	Apples Apricots Cherries Nectarines Papaya Peaches Pears Plum
Eggplant Peppers Mushrooms Potatoes Sweet potato Yams Tomato		Black soy- beans Tempeh Tofu		Corn Green beans Peppers Lentils Olives Potatoes Canned Pump- kin Tomatoes Sweet potato	Cashews
Eggs		Butter Full-fat dairy: Cheese cream milk Sour cream Yogurt		Bananas Cantaloupe Clementine Grapes Honeydew Kiwi Mandarin	

				Orange Pineapple Plantain Raspberry Strawberry Tangelo	
Olives Almonds Almond butter Pistachio Sunflower seed butter Black pepper Vinegars Canned pumpkin Coconut aminos Mustard Pickles Raisins Peppers Tomatoes Raw cruciferous vegetables		Bell peppers Carrots Eggplant Snap peas Snow peas Mushrooms Swiss chard Spinach Tomato		Cold cuts Canned tuna Shellfish Eggs	
		Bullion		Gluten-free bread Gluten-free pasta Almonds	
		Raspberries Strawberries Blackberries honeydew		1 slice wheat bread Biscuits	
		Almonds Nut butters Peanut butter Pistachios Sesame seeds		Bulgur Buckwheat Rice Chips Corn flour Cornflakes Crackers Millet Mixed nuts Oatmeal Oats Peanuts Polenta Popcorn Porridge Potato Flour Pretzels	

				½ cup wheat pasta Rice flour Rice cakes Rice Krispies Sourdough Starch: maize, potato, and tapioca Sorghum Corn chips	
		Sugar-free sweeteners Dark choc-olate		Aspartame Acesulfame K Saccharine Sucralose	
		Paprika Pepper Hot sauce Ketchup Mayonnaise Mustard Olives Pickles Sauerkraut Blue cheese dressing Ranch dress-ing Soy sauce Tomato sauce Vinegars		Chocolate Jam/jelly Ketchup Maple syrup Mayonnaise Mustard Peanut butter Soy sauce Sugar Tomato sauce Vinegars Worcestershire sauce	
				Cheese Lactose-free milk Soy protein Tofu	

RESOURCES

See nmcwellness.com/resources for up to date links and specials for the following products.

Food

Pete's Paleo Chef Prepared Meals—Seasonal & Organic Ingredients—Delivered Fresh

ButcherBox delivers 100% grass-fed beef, free-range organic chicken and heritage breed pork.

Orders through this link will get a $10 off coupon: enter DRTOM10 at checkout.

U.S. Wellness Meats delivers 100% grass-fed and grass-finished beef, lamb, bison, poultry, bone broth, wild-caught seafood

Vital Choice Wild Seafood & Organics fast home delivery of the world's finest wild seafood

Nutritional Supplements

Naturalmedicineformulas.com Highest quality professional line of nutritional supplements. Subscribe and Save.

7-Day Vitamin Box Weekly Pill Organizer, Extra Large Case (7-Day / 4-Times-A-Day)

Kitchen

Cuisinart Steam & Convection Oven

Instant Pot

Excalibur Food Dehydrator

Spiralizer Vegetable Slicer best veggie pasta maker

Vitamix high-speed, professional-grade blender

Face and Body Care

Annmarie Wildcrafted, Organic Skin Care

Dr. Bronner's - Pure-Castile Liquid Soap (Unscented) - Made with Organic Oils

Dr. Bronner's Pure-Castile Bar Soap Made with Organic Oils, For Face and Body

Hair Care

Acure Shampoo and Conditioner Peppermint, Argan Oil & Pumpkin, or Lemongrass. Free of gluten, paraben, sulfate, silicone, phthalate and synthetic fragrance

Oral Care

Dr. Bronner's - All-One Toothpaste (Peppermint) 70% Organic Ingredients, Natural and Effective, Fluoride-Free, SLS-Free, Helps Freshen Breath, Reduce Plaque, Whiten Teeth

Dr. Bronner's - All-One Toothpaste (Cinnamon)

Air Purification

AirDoctor Professional Air Purifier that is 100 times more effective than ordinary HEPA filters

Water Purification

Berkey Water Filter countertop (with optional fluoride filters), shower, sport water bottle

Aquasana Water Filters under the sink, whole house, shower

Infrared Sauna

Clearlight Full Spectrum Infrared Sauna—Low EMF

Fitness

Exercise Ball Professional Grade Balance & Stability Ball

Resistance Bands Exercise Band Set for Working Out

Bosu Balance Trainer for balance, stability, and strength

Medicine Balls for strength and movement exercises

TRX All-in-one Suspension Training: Bodyweight Resistance System. Full Body Workouts for Home

Precor EFX—Elliptical Fitness Crosstrainer:

EFX 221 Home Model

EFX 833 Commercial Model

Beds- Natural, Organic Latex Mattress

Avocado Green Mattress Non-toxic Organic Mattress

EMF Protection

Radiation Free Headphones Earbuds Earphone with Microphone and Volume Control, EMF Protection

REFERENCES

Introduction

Hunter P. (2012). The inflammation theory of disease. The growing realization that chronic inflammation is crucial in many diseases opens new avenues for treatment. *EMBO reports*, 13(11), 968–970. doi:10.1038/embor.2012.142

Pahwa R, Jialal I. Chronic Inflammation. [Updated 2019 Jun 4]. In: StatPearls [Internet]. Treasure Island (FL): StatPearls Publishing; 2019 Jan-. Available from: https://www.ncbi.nlm.nih.gov/books/NBK493173/

Seaman, David R. The diet-induced proinflammatory state: Journal of Manipulative & Physiological Therapeutics, Volume 25, Issue 3, 168 – 179

Seaman, D. R., & Palombo, A. D. (2014). An overview of the identification and management of the metabolic syndrome in chiropractic practice. *Journal of chiropractic medicine*, 13(3), 210–219. doi:10.1016/j.jcm.2014.07.002

Mora, J. R., Iwata, M., & von Andrian, U. H. (2008). Vitamin effects on the immune system: vitamins A and D take centre stage. *Nature reviews. Immunology*, 8(9), 685–698. doi:10.1038/nri2378

Kennedy D. O. (2016). B Vitamins and the Brain: Mechanisms, Dose and Efficacy--A Review. *Nutrients, 8*(2), 68. doi:10.3390/nu8020068

Chapter 1 My Story and How it Can Help You

Zambraski EJ, Rofrano TA, Ciccone CD. Effects of aspirin treatment on kidney function in exercising man. Med Sci Sports Exercise, 1982;14(6):419-23.

Chapter 2 The FreeDiet® Mindset: What is Your Why?

Chapter 3 The FreeDiet® Phase 1

Barclay GR1, McKenzie H, Pennington J, Parratt D, Pennington CR. The effect of dietary yeast on the activity of stable chronic Crohn's disease. Scand J Gastroenterol. 1992;27(3):196-200.

https://kidneystones.uchicago.edu/how-to-eat-a-low-oxalate-diet/

https://www.ewg.org/research/ewgs-good-seafood-guide

https://www.ewg.org/foodnews/summary.php#dirty-dozen

Tournas VH1, Niazi NS2, Kohn JS3. Microbiol Insights. Fungal Presence in Selected Tree Nuts and Dried Fruits. 2015 May 21;8:1-6. doi: 10.4137/MBI.S24308. eCollection 2015.

http://www.sciencetimes.com/articles/13422/20170425/sunflower-seeds-source-toxic-mold-impose-health-risk.htm

Raj Kishor Gupta, Shivraj Singh Gangoliya, and Nand Kumar Singhcorresponding. Reduction of phytic acid and enhancement of bioavailable micronutrients in food grains. J Food Sci Technol. 2015 Feb; 52(2): 676–684. Published online 2013 Apr 24. doi: 10.1007/s13197-013-0978-y

Shi L1, Arntfield SD2, Nickerson M3. Changes in levels of phytic acid, lectins and oxalates during soaking and cooking of Canadian pulses. Food Res Int. 2018 May;107:660-668. doi: 10.1016/j.foodres.2018.02.056. Epub 2018 Mar 5.

V.H.TournasaEugeniaKatsoudasb . Mould and yeast flora in fresh berries, grapes and citrus fruits. International Journal of Food Microbiology. Volume 105, Issue 1, 15 November 2005, Pages 11-17

María L.Fernández-CruzMarcia L.MansillaJosé L.Tadeo. Mycotoxins in fruits and their processed products: Analysis, occurrence and health implications. Journal of Advanced Research Volume 1, Issue 2, April 2010, Pages 113-122

https://www.mayoclinic.org/diseases-conditions/food-allergy/symptoms-causes/syc-20355095

Chapter 4 Overcoming Challenges—How to Stick with it and Succeed

https://aleteia.org/2017/07/12/celiac-disease-does-not-mean-no-eucharist-for-you/

Chapter 5 The FreeDiet® Phase 2

http://static.ewg.org/pdf/US_Gives_Seafood_Eaters_Flawed_Advice_on_Mercury.pdf?_ga=1.191774314.1178297845.1440874084

IgG 21day half-life. Healthscope Functional Pathology Practitioner Manual 2011 p193

Insulin index of foods. http://www.mendosa.com/blog/?p=3624

Chapter 6 The FreeDiet® Phase 3

Oyebode, O., Gordon-Dseagu, V., Walker, A., & Mindell, J. S. (2014). Fruit and vegetable consumption and all-cause, cancer and CVD mortality: analysis of Health Survey for England data. *Journal of epidemiology and community health*, 68(9), 856–862. doi:10.1136/jech-2013-203500

https://wordhistories.net/2017/05/07/one-mans-meat-is-anothers-poison/

Scand J Gastroenterol. 2006 Apr;41(4):408-19.

Drago S1, El Asmar R, Di Pierro M, Grazia Clemente M, Tripathi A, Sapone A, Thakar M, Iacono G, Carroccio A, D'Agate C, Not T, Zampini L, Catassi C, Fasano A. Gliadin, zonulin and gut permeability: Effects on celiac and non-celiac intestinal mucosa and intestinal cell lines. Scand J Gastroenterol. 2006 Apr;41(4):408-19.

Lammers KM1, Lu R, Brownley J, Lu B, Gerard C, Thomas K, Rallabhandi P, Shea-Donohue T, Tamiz A, Alkan S, Netzel-Arnett S, Antalis T, Vogel SN, Fasano A. Gliadin induces an increase in intestinal permeability and zonulin release by binding to the chemokine receptor CXCR3. Gastroenterology. 2008 Jul;135(1):194-204.e3. doi: 10.1053/j.gastro.2008.03.023. Epub 2008 Mar 21.

Seaman, David R. The diet-induced proinflammatory state: Journal of Manipulative & Physiological Therapeutics, Volume 25, Issue 3, 168 – 179

Seaman, D. R., & Palombo, A. D. (2014). An overview of the identification and management of the metabolic syndrome in chiropractic practice. Journal of chiropractic medicine, 13(3), 210–219. doi:10.1016/j.jcm.2014.07.002

Ortiz-Sánchez JP, Cabrera-Chávez F, de la Barca AM. Maize prolamins could induce a gluten-like cellular immune response in some celiac disease patients. *Nutrients*. 2013;5(10):4174–4183. Published 2013 Oct 21. doi:10.3390/nu5104174

Zevallos VF1, Ellis HJ, Suligoj T, Herencia LI, Ciclitira PJ. Variable activation of immune response by quinoa (Chenopodium quinoa Willd.) prolamins in celiac disease. Am J Clin Nutr. 2012 Aug;96(2):337-44. doi: 10.3945/ajcn.111.030684. Epub 2012 Jul 3.

Kennedy L1, Francis H1,2, Alpini G1,2. Fructose Promotion of Intestinal and Liver Injury: A Sugar by Any Other Name That Isn't So Sweet. Hepatology. 2019 Jul 5. doi: 10.1002/hep.30843. [Epub ahead of print]

Lambertz J1, Weiskirchen S1, Landert S2, Weiskirchen R1. Fructose: A Dietary Sugar in Crosstalk with Microbiota Contributing to the Development and Progression of Non-Alcoholic Liver Disease. Front Immunol. 2017 Sep 19;8:1159. doi: 10.3389/fimmu.2017.01159. eCollection 2017.

Mosca A1, Nobili V2, De Vito R3, Crudele A4, Scorletti E5, Villani A6, Alisi A4, Byrne CD5. Serum uric acid concentrations and fructose consumption are independently associated with NASH in children and adolescents. J Hepatol. 2017 May;66(5):1031-1036. doi: 10.1016/j.jhep.2016.12.025. Epub 2017 Feb 14.

Chapter 7 The FreeDiet® Supplements

https://www.nhlbi.nih.gov/health-topics/iron-deficiency-anemia

Zohreh Kheradpisheh,1 Masoud Mirzaei,2 Amir Hossein Mahvi, corresponding author 3,4 Mehdi Mokhtari,1 Reyhane Azizi,5 Hossein Fallahzadeh,6 and Mohammad Hassan Ehrampoush corresponding author1. Impact of Drinking Water Fluoride on Human Thyroid Hormones: A Case-Control Study. Sci Rep. 2018; 8: 2674. Published online 2018 Feb 8.

Adams PC. The modern diagnosis and management of haemochromatosis. Aliment Pharmacol Ther. 2006 Jun 15; 23(12):1681-1691. Review article. PubMed 16817911

de Punder K1, Pruimboom L. The dietary intake of wheat and other cereal grains and their role in inflammation. Nutrients. 2013 Mar 12;5(3):771-87. doi: 10.3390/nu5030771.

Soldin OP. Controversies in urinary iodine determinations. *Clin Biochem.* 2002;35(8):575–579. The diet-induced proinflammatory state: a cause of chronic pain and other degenerative diseases? J Manipulative Physiol Ther. 2002 Mar-Apr;25(3):168-79.

Greenberg JA, Bell SJ. Multivitamin Supplementation During Pregnancy: Emphasis on Folic Acid and l-Methylfolate. Rev Obstet Gynecol. 2011;4(3-4):126–127.

Tafuri L, Servy EJ, Menezo YJ (2018) The hazards of excessive folic acid intake in MTHFR gene mutation carriers: An obstetric and gynecological perspective. Clin Obstet Gynecol Reprod Med 4: doi: 10.15761/COGRM.1000215

Shipton EE, Shipton EA. Vitamin D Deficiency and Pain: Clinical Evidence of Low Levels of Vitamin D and Supplementation in Chronic Pain States. *Pain Ther.* 2015;4(1):67–87. doi:10.1007/s40122-015-0036-8

Helde-Frankling M, Björkhem-Bergman L. Vitamin D in Pain Management. *Int J Mol Sci.* 2017;18(10):2170. Published 2017 Oct 18. doi:10.3390/ijms18102170

Chapter 8 The FreeDiet® Fitness

http://www.stretching-exercises-guide.com/how-long-to-stretch.html

https://fitness.mercola.com/sites/fitness/archive/2010/07/27/the-growing-promise-of-shorter-more-intense-strength-training-workouts.aspx

https://articles.mercola.com/peak-fitness.aspx

Chapter 9 The FreeDiet® Lifestyle—Free for Life

Sears ME, Kerr KJ, Bray RI. Arsenic, cadmium, lead, and mercury in sweat: a systematic review. J Environ Public Health. 2012;2012:184745. doi:10.1155/2012/184745

M Brune, B Magnusson, H Persson, L Hallberg, Iron losses in sweat, The American Journal of Clinical Nutrition, Volume 43, Issue 3, March 1986, Pages 438–443, https://doi.org/10.1093/ajcn/43.3.438

Brewer JH, Thrasher JD, Hooper D. Chronic illness associated with mold and mycotoxins: is naso-sinus fungal biofilm the culprit? Toxins (Basel). 2013;6(1):66–80. Published 2013 Dec 24. doi:10.3390/toxins6010066

Brewer JH1, Thrasher JD, Straus DC, Madison RA, Hooper D. Detection of mycotoxins in patients with chronic fatigue syndrome. Toxins (Basel). 2013 Apr 11;5(4):605-17. doi: 10.3390/toxins5040605

Brewer JH, Thrasher JD, Hooper D. Chronic illness associated with mold and mycotoxins: is naso-sinus fungal biofilm the culprit?. Toxins (Basel). 2013;6(1):66–80. Published 2013 Dec 24. doi:10.3390/toxins6010066

Thrasher JD, Gray MR, Kilburn KH, Dennis DP, Yu A. A water-damaged home and health of occupants: a case study. *J Environ Public Health*. 2012;2012:312836. doi:10.1155/2012/312836

https://www.ewg.org/enviroblog/2011/09/dry-cleaning-chemicals-hang-around-your-clothes

Sherlach, K. S., Gorka, A. P., Dantzler, A. and Roepe, P. D. (2011), Quantification of perchloroethylene residues in dry-cleaned fabrics. Environmental Toxicology and Chemistry, 30: 2481-2487. doi:10.1002/etc.665

Pitts, Connie (2003). "Featured Author. Connie Pitts – Get a Whiff of This: Perfumes (Fragrances) – The Invisible Chemical Poisons."

Anderson RC1, Anderson JH. Acute toxic effects of fragrance products. Arch Environ Health. 1998 Mar-Apr;53(2):138-46.

Anderson RC1, Anderson JH. Toxic effects of air freshener emissions. Arch Environ Health. 1997 Nov-Dec;52(6):433-41.

Kim S1, Hong SH, Bong CK, Cho MH. Characterization of air freshener emission: the potential health effects. J Toxicol Sci. 2015;40(5):535-50. doi: 10.2131/jts.40.535.

Genuis, S. K., Birkholz, D., & Genuis, S. J. (2017). Human Excretion of Polybrominated Diphenyl Ether Flame Retardants: Blood, Urine, and Sweat Study. BioMed research international, 2017, 3676089. doi:10.1155/2017/3676089

Elfide Gizem Kıvrak, Kıymet Kübra Yurt, Arife Ahsen Kaplan, Işınsu Alkan, and Gamze Altun. Effects of electromagnetic fields exposure on the antioxidant defense system. J Microsc Ultrastruct. 2017 Oct-Dec; 5(4): 167–176. Published online 2017 Aug 2. doi:10.1016/j.jmau.2017.07.003

Chapter 10 Next Level Health: Functional & Free™

Li X, Kolltveit KM, Tronstad L, Olsen I. Systemic diseases caused by oral infection. Clin Microbiol Rev. 2000;13(4):547–558. doi:10.1128/cmr.13.4.547-558.2000

Manjunath BC1, Praveen K, Chandrashekar BR, Rani RM, Bhalla A. Periodontal infections: a risk factor for various systemic diseases. Natl Med J India. 2011 Jul-Aug;24(4):214-9.

Patil BS1, Patil S, Gururaj TR. Probable autoimmune causal relationship between periodontitis and Hashimotos thyroidits: a systemic review. Niger J Clin Pract. 2011 Jul-Sep;14(3):253-61. doi: 10.4103/1119-3077.86763.

Admou B, Essaadouni L, Krati K, et al. Atypical celiac disease: from recognizing to managing. Gastroenterol Res Pract. 2012;2012:637187. doi:10.1155/2012/637187

https://ghr.nlm.nih.gov/condition/celiac-disease#genes

Lorini R1, Scaramuzza A, Vitali L, d'Annunzio G, Avanzini MA, De Giacomo C, Severi F. Clinical aspects of coeliac disease in children with insulin-dependent diabetes mellitus. J Pediatr Endocrinol Metab. 1996 Mar;9 Suppl 1:101-11.

Visser J, Rozing J, Sapone A, Lammers K, Fasano A. Tight junctions, intestinal permeability, and autoimmunity: celiac disease and type 1 diabetes paradigms. Ann N Y Acad Sci. 2009;1165:195–205. doi:10.1111/j.1749-6632.2009.04037.x

Aaron Lernera, Torsten Matthiasb. Changes in intestinal tight junction permeability associated with industrial food additives explain the rising incidence of autoimmune disease. Autoimmunity Reviews: Volume 14, Issue 6, June 2015, Pages 479-489

Dr. Alessio Fasano MD, Tarcisio Not MD, Wenle Wang MD, Sergio Uzzau MD, Irene Berti MD, Alberto Tommasini MD, Simeon E Goldblum MD. Zonulin, a newly discovered modulator of intestinal permeability, and its expression in coeliac disease. The Lancet: Volume 355, Issue 9214, 29 April 2000, Pages 1518-1519

Wood RA1. Diagnostic elimination diets and oral food provocation. Chem Immunol Allergy. 2015;101:87-95. doi: 10.1159/000371680. Epub 2015 May 21

Shakoor Z, AlFaifi A, AlAmro B, AlTawil LN, AlOhaly RY. Prevalence of IgG-mediated food intolerance among patients with allergic symptoms. Ann Saudi Med. 2016;36(6):386–390. doi:10.5144/0256-4947.2016.386

Sullivan PB1. Food allergy and food intolerance in childhood. Indian J Pediatr. 1999;66(1 Suppl):S37-45

https://www.elisaact.com/why-eab/our-unique-testing-method/

Beyer K1, Teuber SS. Food allergy diagnostics: scientific and unproven procedures. Curr Opin Allergy Clin Immunol. 2005 Jun;5(3):261-6.

Chapter 11 The FreeDiet® Fix for Thyroid Nodules

Chung H. R. (2014). Iodine and thyroid function. *Annals of pediatric endocrinology & metabolism*, 19(1), 8–12. doi:10.6065/apem.2014.19.1.8

https://www.endocrineweb.com/conditions/thyroid/thyroid-nodules

Barbaro, D., Orrù, B., & Unfer, V. (2019). Iodine and Myo-Inositol: A Novel Promising Combination for Iodine Deficiency. *Frontiers in endocrinology*, 10, 457. doi:10.3389/fendo.2019.00457

Vanderpump MP. Epidemiology of iodine deficiency. Minerva Med. 2017 Apr;108(2):116-123. doi: 10.23736/S0026-4806.16.04918-1. Epub 2016 Dec 14.

Zimmermann MB. Iodine requirements and the risks and benefits of correcting iodine deficiency in populations. J Trace Elem Med Biol. 2008;22(2):81-92. doi: 10.1016/j.jtemb.2008.03.001. Epub 2008 May 7.

Zimmermann MB. Iodine deficiency. Endocr Rev. 2009 Jun;30(4):376-408. doi: 10.1210/er.2009-0011. Epub 2009 May 21.

Dessie G1, Amare D2, Dagnew AB2, Mulugeta H3, Haile Kassa D3, Negesse A4, Kassa GM5, Wagnew F3, Islam SMS6,7, Burrowes S8. Prevalence of goiter among children in Ethiopia and associated factors: a systematic review and meta-analysis. BMC Public Health. 2019 Aug 29;19(1):1191. doi: 10.1186/s12889-019-7505-7.

Chapter 12 The FreeDiet® Fix for Hashimoto's and Autoimmune

Minelli R1, Gaiani F, Kayali S, Di Mario F, Fornaroli F, Leandro G, Nouvenne A, Vincenzi F, De' Angelis GL. Thyroid and celiac disease in pediatric age: a literature review. Acta Biomed. 2018 Dec 17;89(9-S):11-16. doi: 10.23750/abm.v89i9-S.7872.

Spadaccino AC1, Basso D, Chiarelli S, Albergoni MP, D'Odorico A, Plebani M, Pedini B, Lazzarotto F, Betterle C. Celiac disease in North Italian patients with autoimmune thyroid diseases. Autoimmunity. 2008 Feb;41(1):116-21. doi: 10.1080/08916930701620209.

Ch'ng CL1, Biswas M, Benton A, Jones MK, Kingham JG. Prospective screening for coeliac disease in patients with Graves' hyperthyroidism using anti-gliadin and tissue transglutaminase antibodies. Clin Endocrinol (Oxf). 2005 Mar;62(3):303-6.

Janegova A, Janega P1, Rychly B, Kuracinova K, Babal P. The role of Epstein-Barr virus infection in the development of autoimmune thyroid diseases. Endokrynol Pol. 2015;66(2):132-6. doi: 10.5603/EP.2015.0020.

Woodland DL. Epstein-Barr Virus and Grave's Disease. Viral Immunol. 2018 Oct;31(8):539. doi: 10.1089/vim.2018.29031.dlw.

Nagata K, Hara S, Nakayama Y, Higaki K, Sugihara H, Kuwamoto S, Matsushita M, Kato M, Tanio S, Ishiguro K, Hayashi K. Epstein-Barr Virus Lytic Reactivation Induces IgG4 Production by Host B Lymphocytes in Graves' Disease Patients and Controls: A Subset of Graves' Disease Is an IgG4-Related Disease-Like Condition. Viral Immunol. 2018 Oct;31(8):540-547. doi: 10.1089/vim.2018.0042. Epub 2018 Sep 17.

Requena M, López-Villén A, Hernández AF, Parrón T, Navarro Á, Alarcón R. Environmental exposure to pesticides and risk of thyroid diseases. Toxicol Lett. 2019 Aug 21;315:55-63. doi: 10.1016/j.toxlet.2019.08.017.

Tsatsoulis A. The Role of Insulin Resistance/Hyperinsulinism on the Rising Trend of Thyroid and Adrenal Nodular Disease in the Current Environment. J Clin Med. 2018 Feb 26;7(3). pii: E37. doi: 10.3390/jcm7030037.

Köhling HL, Plummer SF, Marchesi JR, Davidge KS, Ludgate M. The microbiota and autoimmunity: Their role in thyroid autoimmune diseases. Clin Immunol. 2017 Oct;183:63-74. doi: 10.1016/j.clim.2017.07.001. Epub 2017 Jul 6.

Wassie MM1,2, Middleton P3,4, Zhou SJ. Agreement between markers of population iodine status in classifying iodine status of populations: a systematic review. Am J Clin Nutr. 2019 Jul 3. pii: nqz118. doi: 10.1093/ajcn/nqz118.

Eman K El-Gayar PhD, Mohamed M Mahmoud. Do protozoa play a role in carcinogenesis? J Egyptian Parasitilogists United. 2014 Vol 7(2): 80-85

Chapter 13 The FreeDiet® Fix for Digestive Issues: IBS and Parasites

Marynowski M, Likońska A, Zatorski H, Fichna J. Role of environmental pollution in irritable bowel syndrome. *World J Gastroenterol.* 2015;21(40):11371–11378. doi:10.3748/wjg.v21.i40.11371

https://articles.mercola.com/sites/articles/archive/2016/11/23/inflammatory-bowel-disease-rise.aspx

Lo Presti, A., Zorzi, F., Del Chierico, F., Altomare, A., Cocca, S., Avola, A., … Guarino, M. (2019). Fecal and Mucosal Microbiota Profiling in Irritable Bowel Syndrome and Inflammatory Bowel Disease. Frontiers in microbiology, 10, 1655. doi:10.3389/fmicb.2019.01655

Nishida, A., Inoue, R., Inatomi, O. et al. Gut microbiota in the pathogenesis of inflammatory bowel disease. Clin J Gastroenterol (2018) 11: 1. https://doi.org/10.1007/s12328-017-0813-5

Serban DE. Microbiota in Inflammatory Bowel Disease Pathogenesis and Therapy: Is It All About Diet? Nutr Clin Pract. 2015 Dec;30(6):760-79. doi: 10.1177/0884533615606898. Epub 2015 Oct 9.

Fritscher-Ravens, Annette et al. Many Patients With Irritable Bowel Syndrome Have Atypical Food Allergies Not Associated With Immunoglobulin E. Gastroenterology, Volume 157, Issue 1, 109 - 118.e5

Chapter 14 The FreeDiet® Fix for Pain

Idris M, Farid J, Gul N. Vitamin D Profile Of Outdoor Patients Presenting With Aches And Pains. J Ayub Med Coll Abbottabad. 2019 Jan-Mar;31(1):51-54.

Geiselman JF. The Clinical Use of IgG Food Sensitivity Testing with Migraine Headache Patients: a Literature Review. Curr Pain Headache Rep. 2019 Aug 27;23(11):79. doi: 10.1007/s11916-019-0819-4.

Peatfield RC. Headache. Relationships between food, wine, and beer-precipitated migrainous headaches. 1995 Jun;35(6):355-7.

Elizabeth Mostofsky, Murray A. Mittleman, Catherine Buettner, Wenyuan Li and Suzanne M. Bertisch, Prospective Cohort Study of Caffeinated Beverage Intake as a Potential Trigger of Headaches among Migraineurs, The American Journal of Medicine, 10.1016/j.amjmed.2019.02.015, (2019).

Brian Edwin Cairns, Influence of pro-algesic foods on chronic pain conditions, Expert Review of Neurotherapeutics, 10.1586/14737175.2016.1157471, 16, 4, (415-423), (2016).

Alessandro Panconesi, Michela Franchini, Maria Letizia Bartolozzi, Stefania Mugnai and Leonello Guidi, Alcoholic Drinks as Triggers in Primary Headaches, Pain Medicine, 14, 8, (1254-1259), (2013).

Taheri, S. (2017). Effect of exclusion of frequently consumed dietary triggers in a cohort of children with chronic primary headache. Nutrition and Health, 23(1), 47–50. https://doi.org/10.1177/0260106016688699

Nilholm, C., Roth, B., & Ohlsson, B. (2019). A Dietary Intervention with Reduction of Starch and Sucrose Leads to Reduced Gastrointestinal and Extra-Intestinal Symptoms in IBS Patients. Nutrients, 11(7), 1662. doi:10.3390/nu11071662

Seaman, David R. The diet-induced proinflammatory state: Journal of Manipulative & Physiological Therapeutics, Volume 25, Issue 3, 168 – 179

Seaman, D. R., & Palombo, A. D. (2014). An overview of the identification and management of the metabolic syndrome in chiropractic practice. Journal of chiropractic medicine, 13(3), 210–219. doi:10.1016/j.jcm.2014.07.002

Chapter 15 The FreeDiet® Fix for Fatigue and Brain Fog

Wolffenbuttel, B., Wouters, H., Heiner-Fokkema, M. R., & van der Klauw, M. M. (2019). The Many Faces of Cobalamin (Vitamin B12) Deficiency. Mayo Clinic proceedings. Innovations, quality & outcomes, 3(2), 200–214. doi:10.1016/j.mayocpiqo.2019.03.002

https://www.medicinenet.com/chronic_fatigue_syndrome/article.htm#chronic_fatigue_syndrome_cfs_or_systemic_exertion_intolerance_disease_seid_facts

Pavlov CS1, Damulin IV1, Shulpekova YO1, Andreev EA. Neurological disorders in vitamin B12 deficiency. Ter Arkh. 2019 May 16;91(4):122-129. doi: 10.26442/00403660.2019.04.000116.

Darling KA, Eggleston MJF, Retallick-Brown H, Rucklidge JJ. Mineral-Vitamin Treatment Associated with Remission in Attention-Deficit/Hyperactivity Disorder Symptoms and Related Problems: 1-Year Naturalistic Outcomes of a 10-Week Randomized Placebo-Controlled Trial. J Child Adolesc Psychopharmacol. 2019 Jul 25. doi: 10.1089/cap.2019.0036.

Rucklidge JJ, Eggleston MJF, Johnstone JM, Darling K, Frampton CM. Vitamin-mineral treatment improves aggression and emotional regulation in children with ADHD: a fully blinded, randomized, placebo-controlled trial. J Child Psychol Psychiatry. 2018 Mar;59(3):232-246. doi: 10.1111/jcpp.12817.

Rucklidge, J. J., Frampton, C. M., Gorman, B., & Boggis, A. (2017). Vitamin–Mineral Treatment of ADHD in Adults: A 1-Year Naturalistic Follow-Up of a Randomized Controlled Trial. Journal of Attention Disorders, 21(6), 522–532. https://doi.org/10.1177/1087054714530557

Wurzinger B1, König P [Iron deficiency, Fatigue and Restless-Legs-Syndrome].[Article in German] Wien Med Wochenschr. 2016 Oct;166(13-14):447-452. Epub 2016 Aug 30.

Fehr J1, Favrat B, Schleiffenbaum B, Krayenbühl PA, Kapanci C, von Orelli F. [Diagnosis and treatment of iron deficiency without anaemia]. [Article in German]. Praxis (Bern 1994). 2009 Dec 2;98(24):1445-51. doi: 10.1024/1661-8157.98.24.1445.

DeLoughery TG. Iron Deficiency Anemia. Med Clin North Am. 2017 Mar;101(2):319-332. doi: 10.1016/j.mcna.2016.09.004. Epub 2016 Dec 8.

Skjellerudsveen, B. M., Omdal, R., & Grimstad, T. (2019). Fatigue in celiac disease: A review of the literature. JGH open : an open access journal of gastroenterology and hepatology, 3(3), 242–248. doi:10.1002/jgh3.12134

Busby, E., Bold, J., Fellows, L., & Rostami, K. (2018). Mood Disorders and Gluten: It's Not All in Your Mind! A Systematic Review with Meta-Analysis. Nutrients, 10(11), 1708. doi:10.3390/nu10111708

Peters SL1, Biesiekierski JR, Yelland GW, Muir JG, Gibson PR. Randomised clinical trial: gluten may cause depression in subjects with non-coeliac gluten sensitivity - an exploratory clinical study. Aliment Pharmacol Ther. 2014 May;39(10):1104-12. doi: 10.1111/apt.12730. Epub 2014 Apr 1.

Chapter 16 The FreeDiet® Fix for Fat

Hills, R. D., Jr, Pontefract, B. A., Mishcon, H. R., Black, C. A., Sutton, S. C., & Theberge, C. R. (2019). Gut Microbiome: Profound Implications for Diet and Disease. Nutrients, 11(7), 1613. doi:10.3390/nu11071613

Jönsson, T., Memon, A. A., Sundquist, K., Sundquist, J., Olsson, S., Nalla, A., … Linse, S. (2015). Digested wheat gluten inhibits binding between leptin and its receptor. BMC biochemistry, 16, 3. doi:10.1186/s12858-015-0032-y

You, W., & Henneberg, M. (2016). Cereal Crops Are not Created Equal: Wheat Consumption Associated with Obesity Prevalence Globally and Regionally. AIMS public health, 3(2), 313–328. doi:10.3934/publichealth.2016.2.313

Roccisano, D. Henneberg, M. Soy consumption and obesity. Food and Nutrition Sciences, 2012; 3(2):260-266

Weeratunga, P., Jayasinghe, S., Perera, Y., Jayasena, G., & Jayasinghe, S. (2014). Per capita sugar consumption and prevalence of diabetes mellitus--global and regional associations. BMC public health, 14, 186. doi:10.1186/1471-2458-14-186

Garduño-Alanís A, Malyutina S, Pajak A, Stepaniak U, Kubinova R, Denisova D, Pikhart H, Peasey A, Bobak M, Stefler D. Association between soft drink, fruit juice consumption and obesity in Eastern Europe: cross-sectional and longitudinal analysis of the HAPIEE study. J Hum Nutr Diet. 2019 Sep 1. doi: 10.1111/jhn.12696.

Dubois, Lise et al. Regular Sugar-Sweetened Beverage Consumption between Meals Increases Risk of Overweight among Preschool-Aged Children. Journal of the American Dietetic Association, Volume 107, Issue 6, 924 - 934

Bueno NB1, de Melo IS, de Oliveira SL, da Rocha Ataide T. Very-low-carbohydrate ketogenic diet v. low-fat diet for long-term weight loss: a meta-analysis of randomised controlled trials. Br J Nutr. 2013 Oct;110(7):1178-87. doi: 10.1017/S0007114513000548. Epub 2013 May 7.

Clifton PM1, Bastiaans K, Keogh JB. High protein diets decrease total and abdominal fat and improve CVD risk profile in overweight and obese men and women with elevated triacylglycerol. Nutr Metab Cardiovasc Dis. 2009 Oct;19(8):548-54. doi: 10.1016/j.numecd.2008.10.006. Epub 2009 Jan 29.

Goday, A., Bellido, D., Sajoux, I., Crujeiras, A. B., Burguera, B., García-Luna, P. P., … Casanueva, F. F. (2016). Short-term safety, tolerability and efficacy of a very low-calorie-ketogenic diet interventional weight loss program versus hypocaloric diet in patients with type 2 diabetes mellitus. Nutrition & diabetes, 6(9), e230. doi:10.1038/nutd.2016.36

Chapter 17 The FreeDiet® Fix for High Ferritin

VanWagner LB, Green RM. Elevated serum ferritin. JAMA. 2014;312(7):743–744. doi:10.1001/jama.2014.302

Goot K1, Hazeldine S, Bentley P, Olynyk J, Crawford D. Elevated serum ferritin - what should GPs know? Aust Fam Physician. 2012 Dec;41(12):945-9.

Swinkels DW1, Marx JJ. [Diagnosis and treatment of primary hemochromatosis]. Ned Tijdschr Geneeskd. 1999 Jul 3;143(27):1404-8.

Horváth G1, Dávid K. Iron storage disease. Orv Hetil. 2004 Sep 26;145(39):1979-84.

Kelley, M., Joshi, N., Xie, Y., & Borgaonkar, M. (2014). Iron overload is rare in patients homozygous for the H63D mutation. Canadian journal of gastroenterology & hepatology, 28(4), 198–202.

Samarasena J, Winsor W, Lush R, Duggan P, Xie Y, Borgaonkar M. Individuals homozygous for the H63D mutation have significantly elevated iron indexes. Dig Dis Sci. 2006 Apr;51(4):803-7.

Chapter 18 The FreeDiet® Fix for High Blood Pressure

http://www.onlinejacc.org/content/71/19/e127?_
ga=2.230084890.729625539.1556377593-1710169387.1556377593

https://www.heart.org/-/media/data-import/downloadables/hypertension-guideline-highlights-flyer-ucm_497841.pdf

https://onlinelibrary.wiley.com/doi/full/10.1111/j.1751-7176.2011.00489.x

https://onlinelibrary.wiley.com/doi/abs/10.1002/jmv.24391

Houston M1. The role of magnesium in hypertension and cardiovascular disease. J Clin Hypertens (Greenwich). 2011 Nov;13(11):843-7. doi: 10.1111/j.1751-7176.2011.00538.x. Epub 2011 Sep 26.

Champagne CM. Magnesium in hypertension, cardiovascular disease, metabolic syndrome, and other conditions: a review. Nutr Clin Pract. 2008 Apr-May;23(2):142-51. doi: 10.1177/0884533608314533.

He K, Liu K, Daviglus ML, Morris SJ, Loria CM, Van Horn L, Jacobs DR Jr, Savage PJ. Magnesium intake and incidence of metabolic syndrome among young adults. Circulation. 2006 Apr 4;113(13):1675-82. Epub 2006 Mar 27.

Chapter 19 The FreeDiet® Recipes

https://spoonfulofhealth.com/category/freediet-phase-1/

https://www.ewg.org/foodnews/summary.php#dirty-dozen

Appendix

https://thepaleodiet.com

https://autoimmunewellness.com for the AIP diet

https://www.thecandidadiet.com

https://www.bulletproof.com

https://bodyecology.com

https://www.precisionnutrition.com/elimination-diet

https://www.dietdoctor.com for the Keto diet

https://www.monashfodmap.com

https://whole30.com

ABOUT THE AUTHOR

Dr. Tom Rofrano is the founder and director of the Natural Medicine Clinic in Palm Beach Gardens, Florida and has successfully seen over 100,000 patient visits during the past 33+ years.

He has studied health and nutrition since age 12 on a lifelong quest to heal from his many ailments. Even though his father was a medical doctor and his mother a nurse, he was frequently sick and injured. While traditional medicine and diets failed, he was able to free himself from Hashimoto's thyroid disease, rheumatoid arthritis, gout, peripheral neuropathy, IBS, and other health conditions.

Through detailed evaluation and testing as a chiropractic physician and functional medicine practitioner, he helps patients discover their root cause and provides them with clear solutions to get better.

Through many years of experience with patients and on his quest for healing, he developed the FreeDiet® and has helped thousands free themselves from gut and thyroid issues, pain, fatigue, autoimmune, and other chronic health conditions so they can enjoy their lives again.

You can visit him online at drtomrofrano.com.

Made in the USA
Las Vegas, NV
16 June 2021

24763945R00132